Stop
Stress
This Minute

Editorial Staff

Author: James Porter

Executive Editor: David Hunnicutt, PhD

Managing Editor: Brittanie Leffelman, MS

Contributing Editor: Madeline Jahn, MOL

Multimedia Designer: Adam Paige

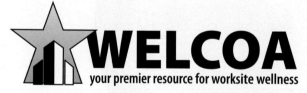

WELCOA
your premier resource for worksite wellness

17002 Marcy Street, Suite 140 | Omaha, NE 68118
PH: 402-827-3590 | FX: 402-827-3594 | welcoa.org

Table of Contents

About **WELCOA**

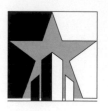

The Wellness Council of America (WELCOA) was established as a national not-for-profit organization in the mid 1980s through the efforts of a number of forward-thinking business and health leaders. Drawing on the vision originally set forth by William Kizer, Sr., Chairman Emeritus of Central States Indemnity, and WELCOA founding Directors that included Dr. Louis Sullivan, former Secretary of Health and Human Services, and Warren Buffet, Chairman of Berkshire Hathaway, WELCOA has helped influence the face of workplace wellness in the US.

Today, WELCOA has become one of the most respected resources for workplace wellness in America. With a membership in excess of 5,000 organizations, WELCOA is dedicated to improving the health and well-being of all working Americans. Located in America's heartland, WELCOA makes its national headquarters in one of America's healthiest business communities—Omaha, Nebraska.

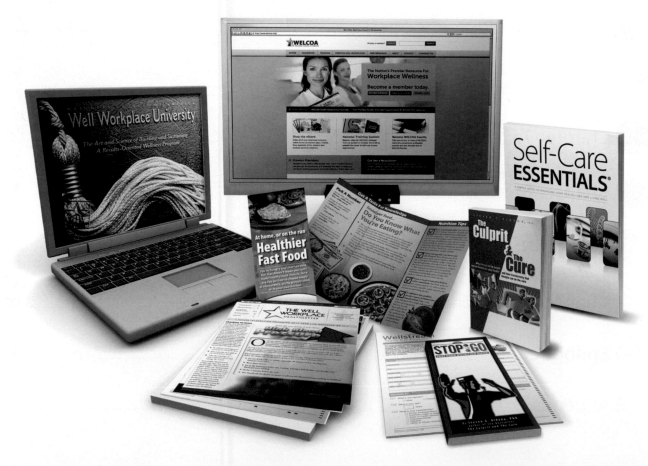

About **James Porter**

James E. Porter is president of StressStop.com, a company that has been providing stress management training materials to corporations, hospitals, government agencies and military bases for over 20 years. Mr. Porter is the author and creator of many of these materials which include workbooks, DVDs, CDs, dozens of articles, and a weekly blog on stress management.

His work has been reviewed and/or reported on in major news outlets including *Good Morning America, Ladies Home Journal, The Associated Press, WCBS-TV News* and *The NY Daily News*, as well as in medical journals including *The Journal of Family Practice, The Journal of Cardiopulmonary Rehabilitation*, and *The Journal of Biomedical Communications*.

Mr. Porter's video programs can be seen over CC-TV in thousands of hospitals nationwide, including The Mayo Clinic, The Cleveland Clinic and at the Mind/Body Clinic in Boston, Mass. His workbook, *The Stress Profiler*, has sold over 250,000 copies. Dr. Albert Ellis, cofounder of the cognitive branch of psychology, called his DVD *Short Circuiting Stress*, "a remarkably clear and useful self-help video."

Mr. Porter has also presented stress management seminars onsite for *Time, Inc, Glaxo Smith Kline, Blue Cross Blue Shield, The Department of Homeland Security, The FBI, The American Heart Association, The International Stress Management Association, The Navy, The Marines*, and *The Army*. He is a Fellow of The American Institute of Stress. You can find out more about managing stress at his website: **www.StressStop.com**

FOREWORD

Countdown To
Serenity

There's no question that stress is epidemic in the western world. It has been estimated that over two-thirds of office visits to physicians are for stress-related illnesses and concerns. Stress is a major contributing factor to the six leading causes of death in the United States—either directly or indirectly impacting coronary artery disease, cancer, respiratory disorders, accidental injuries, cirrhosis of the liver and suicide. What's more, stress aggravates other conditions such as multiple sclerosis, diabetes, mental illness, alcoholism and drug abuse, and if left unchecked, it can fuel family discord and violence.

Sadly, the stress epidemic is an extremely costly one. The medical costs are estimated to be in the billions of dollars per year in the US alone. In addition, stress impacts business and industry to the tune of approximately 150 billion dollars per year in increased health insurance outlays, burnout, absenteeism and reduced productivity, costly mistakes in the office and on the shop floor, poor morale and high employee turnover.

Relentless stress takes its toll in the lives of American workers in a variety of ways. Both additive and cumulative, stress adds up over time until a state of crisis is reached and symptoms appear. These symptoms may manifest themselves psychologically as irritability, anxiety, impaired concentration, mental confusion, poor judgment, frustration and anger. Stress may also appear in the additional manifestation of physical symptoms. Common physical symptoms of stress include: muscle tension, headaches, low back pain, insomnia and high blood pressure. If left untreated, these symptoms may lead to physical illness and sometimes disability and death.

But what's perhaps most interesting about stress is that it has both positive and negative implications in the lives of working Americans. Properly harnessed good stress—known as eustress—can motivate us and allow us to accomplish extraordinary things. On the other hand, negative stress—also known as distress—is what brings us to our knees.

In this remarkable book, one of the nation's best stress experts provides a step-by-step blueprint that will help you stop your stress this minute. Edited by Madeline Jahn, this book is written in a simple and straightforward format that's fully-illustrated. It's designed to be one of those rare tools that can provide you with the instruction you need to not only manage stress, but to conquer it completely. There's no other book on the market quite like it. And, if you follow the recommendations and instruction set forth in the following pages, you'll be a better person—happier, healthier and more productive.

In closing, I'd like to thank Jim Porter for making this important contribution in helping all working Americans and their families to lead healthier lives—this book is going to become a standard in workplaces throughout the US. My advice to you is to read it from cover to cover. Meditate on the advice—roll it over in your mind. Ultimately, I challenge you to put the principles to good use in your life. The outcome will be nothing short of remarkable.

Yours in good health,

D. Hunnicutt

David Hunnicutt, PhD
President
Wellness Council of America

ABOUT DR. DAVID HUNNICUTT

Since his arrival at WELCOA in 1995, David Hunnicutt, PhD has developed countless publications that have been widely adopted in businesses and organizations throughout North America. Known for his ability to make complex issues easier to understand, David has a proven track-record of publishing health and wellness material that helps employees lead healthier lifestyles. David travels extensively advocating better health practices and radically different thinking in organizations of all kinds.

CHAPTER 1

What Is Your Stress Number?

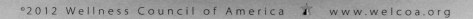

CHAPTER 1

What Is Your Stress Number?

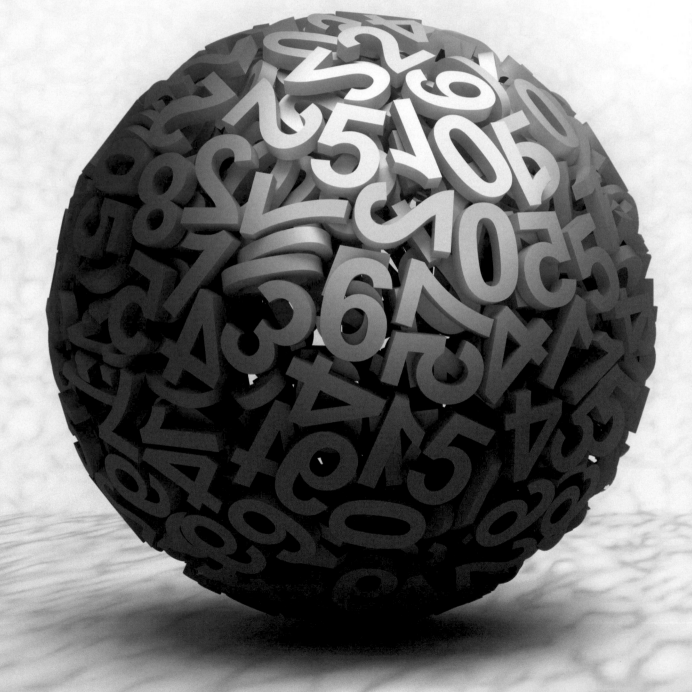

Stress is everywhere you look: It's in the little things that get under your skin such as traffic jams, difficult customers, long lines, rude remarks, bad drivers, noisy neighbors and impolite children. It's in the bigger things that drag you down, such as downsizing, rising prices, unemployment, angry bosses, having to work two jobs, crime, terrorism and even foreign wars. And then there are those life-changing events, such as accidents, illness, the death of a loved one, getting laid-off, or going through a divorce or breakup. These are just a few of the stressful influences that leave us feeling sad, anxious, nervous, frustrated, frightened, overwhelmed, depressed, lonely and/or just plain lousy.

How Do We Manage This Ever Increasing Stressload?

Typically, we "manage" our stress by overspending, overeating, smoking, drinking and even becoming dependent on prescription and over-the-counter drugs like pain killers and sleeping pills. Also known as "counter-productive coping," this way of handling stress only leads to even bigger problems such as maxed-out credit cards, obesity, diabetes, lung cancer and alcoholism—which only adds fuel to the fire.

Experts estimate that between 75 to 90% of all doctors visits are for stress-related conditions. (Maybe you've experienced some of these stress-related conditions yourself?) They include: migraine headaches, tension headaches, colitis, irritable bowel syndrome, fibromyalgia, chronic fatigue, asthma, allergies, rashes, anxiety, depression, insomnia and back pain. These conditions can all be adversely affected by stress.

"Prescriptive Solutions" Don't Get To The Heart Of The Problem

Doctors are sometimes as baffled as their patients by the reason for the symptoms—so they quickly prescribe any pills that might temporarily lessen their patient's pain. But these "prescriptive" solutions often come with a price (AKA side effects), which, depending on the prescription offered, may or may not include: drowsiness, weight gain, agitation, low libido, lethargy and—in rare cases—death.

Besides some pretty scary side effects, there's another big problem with this pharmacological approach. When you take a sleeping pill, a pain pill, an anti-anxiety drug like Xanax or Valium—you're usually not addressing the *source* of the problem. You're eliminating the symptom, but not the cause of the symptom.

> "Experts estimate that between 75 to 90% of all doctors visits are for stress-related conditions."

Of course you can make it easier to cope with the problem by eliminating or reducing these annoying symptoms like sleeplessness, pain, nervousness and low mood. But, you are absolutely NOT addressing the root of the problem. The pharmacological approach is roughly the equivalent of asking your auto-mechanic to put masking tape over a warning light on the dashboard of your car. Your problem isn't fixed, you're just not as aware of it anymore.

Doctors write out most prescriptions for a limited time. They hope the prescription will get you through a rough patch, and that when it runs out, you won't need it any more. That's the hope. But when the rough patch doesn't go away for weeks, months or years, then what do you do? If you're like most people, you go back to your doctor and ask (and in some cases beg) for the prescription to be renewed. And, as a result, your body continues to take a beating while you carefully cover up all the evidence (or symptoms) of your stress. In effect, you're pharmacologically propping yourself up, acting as if you have no symptoms.

> "This book is about how to get you out of a vicious cycle you may not even know you are in."

As you can see, there are some fundamental flaws with this approach to handling stress. We either make our problems worse by overeating, over-spending or over-drinking—or we try to cover them up with a pill that may or may not be good for us in the long run.

With options like these, *something has to change.*

This Book Is About Helping You Make That Change

This book is about how to get you out of a vicious cycle you may not even know you are in. All the solutions (mostly counter-productive) that have been mentioned so far—from overeating to over-drinking to over-dependence on prescription drugs—only anesthetize you to the pain. They allow you to keep going when your body is screaming for you to stop!

You say to yourself: *"If I just keep on pushing myself, maybe I'll get through this rough patch."* This book is also about how to address what's causing the rough patch. It's about understanding the rough patch, finding all-natural ways of getting through the rough patch, and what to do when the rough patch doesn't go away.

Managing stress is not as hard as you think. In fact, *you can lower your stress right now.* Not next week, or next month or even next year, *but right this minute.* And you won't need a pill or a drink, or even have to pull out your wallet to do it.

www.welcoa.org ⭐ ©2012 Wellness Council of America

Are You Interested?

If so, start by ranking your stress (how tense or relaxed you feel right now) on a scale from zero to ten. Zero is the complete absence of tension, (no anxious feelings in the gut or tension in the body), and 10 is a full-blown panic attack, (where you have so much tension that you either feel like you are having heart-attack-like symptoms, tunnel vision, feeling sweaty all over, or are having a nervous breakdown.)

So what's your stress number right now? Write it in the box to the right. (Don't over-think this. A reasonable guess is fine.)

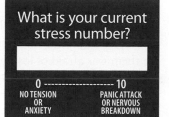

What is your current stress number?

0 -------------------- 10
NO TENSION OR ANXIETY · PANIC ATTACK OR NERVOUS BREAKDOWN

Look at your watch or a clock. Before the second hand goes around twice, you are going to significantly lower your level of stress and by so doing, learn to self-regulate your nervous-system. Here's how.

HOW TO SELF-REGULATE YOUR NERVOUS SYSTEM

Take a minute to reflect on the following instructions before beginning.

- ⏱ **Breathe in deeply (through your nose) to a count of four.**
- ⏱ **Hold that breath in for a count of four.**
- ⏱ **And then, breathe out to a count of six.**
- ⏱ **Repeat this cycle three times.**

Reread these instructions until you have them memorized. Close your eyes if desired before beginning. (Please do the above breathing exercise before continuing on.)

What is your stress number now?

If you're second number is lower than your first, then you've just done something that Western science once thought was impossible. You've self-regulated your autonomic nervous system.

About The Autonomic Nervous System

It's called the autonomic nervous system (or ANS for short) because it's supposed to work on auto-pilot, without any conscious control by you. Up until the 1960s, most Western scientists believed you couldn't self-regulate your autonomic nervous system. Then, in the late-sixties, a group of yoga practitioners agreed to meet at a lab on the campus of Harvard University to see if they could control the ANS by simply meditating. This idea was considered so radical at the time that the Harvard professor who had agreed to see them was afraid of losing his job. That's why he had his test subjects meet him at night—he wanted to minimize any chances of his colleagues finding out what he was doing. That professor's name was Dr. Herbert Benson.

In his lab, and later in his writing, Dr. Benson would identify the antidote to what we now refer to as *the fight or flight response*. (But more about Dr. Benson later.)

The Fight Or Flight Response

The fight or flight response was a term coined by another professor at Harvard, Dr. Walter Cannon, (as it turns out, in the very same lab) fifty years earlier. His research explained why our hearts beat faster, our pupils dilate, our blood vessels constrict, our mouth dries up and our muscles become tense whenever we experience stress. Cannon theorized that this response allowed our prehistoric ancestors to go from a calm state to a highly aroused state in a matter of seconds, and that it had evolved over millions of years.

These fast-acting physiological changes of the fight or flight response were designed to help our prehistoric ancestors fight an attacker or flee to safety, hence its name. This response worked perfectly for the caveman who used it only when his life was in danger. However, in our modern world, this primitive response tends to backfire. Our stressors today consist mostly of psychological threats to our well-being, such as a rude remark, a car honk or a bad day at the office. None of these stressors could possibly kill us, but we react to them as *if they could*—almost like the caveman would react to the sight of a lion or a tiger.

"Managing stress is not as hard as you think. In fact, you can lower your stress right now. Not next week, or next month or even next year, but right this minute. And you won't need a pill or a drink, or even have to pull out your wallet to do it."

When you find yourself in a stressful situation and you hear yourself saying "I'd like to strangle that guy," or "I'm really angry with him or her," or "I'm not going to take this anymore," you probably have already *needlessly* activated your fight or flight response. When you feel your hands get cold and clammy before getting up to put on a presentation, you have already *needlessly* activated your fight or flight response. When you feel your heart pounding when someone cuts ahead of you in line, you have already *needlessly* activated your fight or flight response.

Why is it needless? Because in all of these modern-day situations you're basically stuck: *You can't fight and you can't flee.* This response does you absolutely no good at all. *In fact, this same response that was designed to save our prehistoric ancestors is gradually (and in some cases, not so gradually) killing us now.* It's needlessly calling up all this energy and tension, for which there is no outlet and no purpose. This puts a lot of unnecessary wear and tear on the body that eventually shows up in the form of pain or disease.

The Harmful Effects Of Too Much Stress

When you see the connection between your strong reactions and the events that precede them you begin to realize the power that this stress response has over us. And when we look at the changes that take place during fight or flight, it becomes painfully obvious that there's a connection between what the stress response does to the body and the list of stress-related diseases to which it can lead.

Think about that word disease for a moment and break it down into two syllables. DIS-EASE. *It's a synonym for the word stress!* (See the list of stress-related diseases in the sidebar.)

The fight or flight response fills us full of adrenaline, raises our blood pressure, causes our hearts to beat faster, shuts down our immune system, halts our digestive system, turns off our reproductive system and even causes our bowels and bladder to "void," all in an effort to make us into a lean, mean fighting (or fleeing) machine. Is it any wonder then, that insomnia, high blood pressure, heart disease, immune system disorders, infertility and digestive tract disorders are the most common types of stress-related concerns? Do you see the relationship between what the fight or flight response does to our body and why (when we activate it chronically and unnecessarily) it makes us sick?

Dr. Martin Samuels has an interesting job. He is head of the Neuro-Cardiology Department at Brigham and Women's Hospital in Boston, Massachusetts, where he studies the relationship between THINKING and heart-disease.

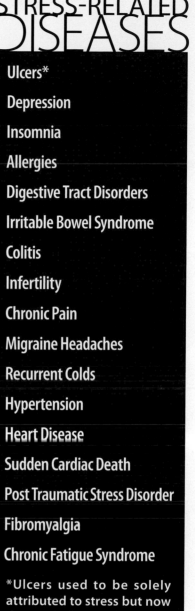

STRESS-RELATED DISEASES

Ulcers*

Depression

Insomnia

Allergies

Digestive Tract Disorders

Irritable Bowel Syndrome

Colitis

Infertility

Chronic Pain

Migraine Headaches

Recurrent Colds

Hypertension

Heart Disease

Sudden Cardiac Death

Post Traumatic Stress Disorder

Fibromyalgia

Chronic Fatigue Syndrome

*Ulcers used to be solely attributed to stress but now they are believed to be caused by the helicobacter pylori bacterium. Yet most people (80%) have this bacterium in their gut all the time. Still, only a small percentage of these EVER develop ulcers. Stress experts suggest that maybe stress makes the gut more vulnerable to the bacteria and that's why the ulcer develops.

Scared To Death?

One of Dr. Samuels' work-related hobbies is collecting stories of otherwise healthy people who were literally scared to death. Ken Lay, the CEO of ENRON—who died suddenly of a heart attack while awaiting sentencing—may have been an example of someone who was scared to death. Samuels has also collected several stories of young people with absolutely no history of heart disease who died suddenly while riding a roller coaster. He even has evidence of several medically-confirmed accounts of voodoo death where the victims' strong belief in the power of the medicine man was enough to kill them.

All of these examples attest to the extraordinary power of the autonomic nervous system (ANS.) "The ANS uses the hormone adrenaline, a neurotransmitter, or chemical messenger, to send signals to various parts of the body to activate the fight-or-flight response," Dr. Samuels explained in an interview in *Scientific American*. "This chemical is toxic in large amounts; it damages the internal organs such as the heart, lungs, liver and kidneys. It is believed that almost all sudden deaths are caused by damage to the heart."

Triggering Stress Hormones

Another neurotransmitter related to the stress response is called cortisol. Cortisol is the stress hormone that makes you feel tense, irritable and edgy. It rises and falls throughout the day. It's typically highest in the morning when you wake up and lowest at night when you go to sleep. But it can rise and fall during the day for other reasons, such as when you are late for work and get stuck in a traffic jam. It can also rise when you drink caffeinated beverages such as coffee, tea or cola.

You can even make your cortisol levels rise by simply *thinking* of something stressful. For instance, I have a picture of a rock climber next to my desk. He climbs with no equipment, ropes or grappling hooks and hangs from a hundred foot cliff with his bare hands. All I have to do is LOOK at that picture and my cortisol levels rise. As for the recipient of a voodoo spell, or Ken Lay, or the kids on the rollercoaster—their *thoughts* resulted in a drenching of stress-hormones that led to death. Even though those kinds of fatal events are very rare, stress is NOT something that you should underestimate or take lightly.

Many stress experts believe that much of the degenerative illnesses we suffer from today are the result of our organs being bathed in high levels of stress hormones throughout the day. Even after a minor stressful episode, it usually takes about 40 minutes for your stress hormones to return to normal. But if you have more stressful events within that same time frame, the stress hormones in your body cascade one level on top of another until you often just blow your top.

> "The ANS (autonomic nervous system) uses the hormone adrenaline, a neurotransmitter, or chemical messenger, to send signals to various parts of the body to activate the fight-or-flight response."

> "Even after a minor stressful episode, it usually takes about 40 minutes for your stress hormones to return to normal. But if you have more stressful events within that same time frame, the stress hormones in your body cascade one level on top of another until you often just blow your top."

The Importance Of Monitoring Your Stress Number

It's your stress hormones fluctuating throughout the day that give you that subtle feeling of anxiety in the pit of your stomach. When you wake up and realize today's the day you are having a root canal, both your level of stress hormones and your stress number are going to rise. However, when you stop to rank your stress on a scale from 0-10, to a large degree, you are self-monitoring your stress hormones.

And by so doing, you are giving yourself the opportunity to stop your stress from getting *out of control*. Stressful events can and do build on previous stressful events. And when you lose control in regrettable ways, it's usually the result of a progression of stressful events and not one isolated incident.

(Even though, through lack of awareness, you may think it was only the ONE straw that broke the camel's back.) When you take the time to monitor your stress levels, you will learn some interesting lessons.

The Mianus River Bridge Lesson

A lesson I learned while driving on Interstate 95 over the Mianus River Bridge in Greenwich, CT, helped me forever change the way I think about and ultimately manage my stress—and I believe it will do the same for you.

First, a little background about the Mianus River Bridge: On June 28, 1983 the bridge collapsed in the middle of the night without any warning. The timing was lucky because only three people died. If it had collapsed in the daytime, the death toll would have been much higher. About 100,000 cars a day passed over that bridge at the time. I lived in Greenwich back then and even drove over that bridge on the day it collapsed.

Fast-forward twenty years to 2003.
I was then living in a town about ten miles up the road and I rarely went over that bridge. But when I did, for some reason, it was beginning to frighten me. Whenever I would meet an old friend to play tennis in Greenwich, I could feel my anxiety levels grow from about a four to a seven in the half mile or so it took to cross over the bridge. Just when it felt like I was about to have a panic attack, I'd reach the other side and my stress would subside.

But here's the most interesting (and at first, baffling) part of all: on my return trip I would feel no anxiety crossing the bridge what-so-ever! What was going on? How could I have almost had a panic attack in one direction and not feel a thing in the other. It took several trips—and the very same stress number technique I'm teaching you—to figure it out.

Here's what I determined: On the way down, I was stressed. I was in a hurry. I didn't want to be late. I was driving in rush hour traffic. And I was inherently (and with probable cause) just a little afraid of that bridge. Add to this volatile mix of stress chemicals the jolt of adrenaline I'd feel from just ANTICIPATING a competitive game of tennis—and there you have it.

I'd start out on the north side of that bridge bathing in cortisol and adrenaline and my stress number would already be at a five when I arrived at the bridge. By the time I got over to the other side, heart pumping with anxiety, my stress level and therefore, stress number, had cumulatively built on the stress chemicals ALREADY in my system and would often reach as high as a seven.

However, on the south side of that bridge—coming back—my stress number would start out much lower. The reason? My friend and I would have played about an hour or two of tennis. I would be exhausted from physical exertion. We'd always relax, laugh and have a good time afterwards. My exercise endorphins (the body's own morphine) would kick in, and on the way back—since it wasn't rush hour and I wasn't in a hurry—I'd hit the bridge from the south side with my stress number at a zero or a one. Thus, any elevation in my stress levels that occurred while I was actually on the bridge would barely even be noticeable.

> Much of our stress is cumulative and major stressful events usually don't happen out of the blue. Often times, it's a cascading series of events, the first couple of which might be too minor to even notice. But as these events build, so do the stress hormones in your body, and so does the likelihood of you getting even more stressed.

This dichotomy between the going over and the coming home was a real eye-opener for me. I realized that MANY of the stressful situations in my life were only intolerable because I went into them feeling stressed ahead of time. And, if I could somehow keep track of and lower my stress beforehand, these so-called intolerably stressful events would have been much less stressful and sometimes not stressful at all!

I have applied this insight to all kinds of situations—whether flying on a plane, speaking in public, or going to see the dentist. Any stressful situation that I can *anticipate ahead of time,* I can now control by simply bringing my stress number down to zero or one beforehand, using techniques like the ones we'll demonstrate in Chapter 2.

Stress Is Cumulative

This is probably the most important thing I've EVER learned about stress: much of our stress is cumulative and major stressful events usually don't happen out of the blue. Often times, it's a cascading series of events, the first couple of which might be too minor to even notice. But as these events build, so do the stress hormones in your body, and so does the likelihood of you getting even more stressed.

And even more importantly, I learned that you can control your stress by simply tracking your stress levels at all times, but especially before the start of something you KNOW is going to be stressful like going to the dentist or going on a job interview. ⏱

We have already shattered one myth about stress management. Do you know what it is? If so, write it down.

....

....

....

....

Hint: It's something that Western Scientists didn't believe you could do.

CHAPTER 2

Self-Regulating Your Nervous System

www.welcoa.org

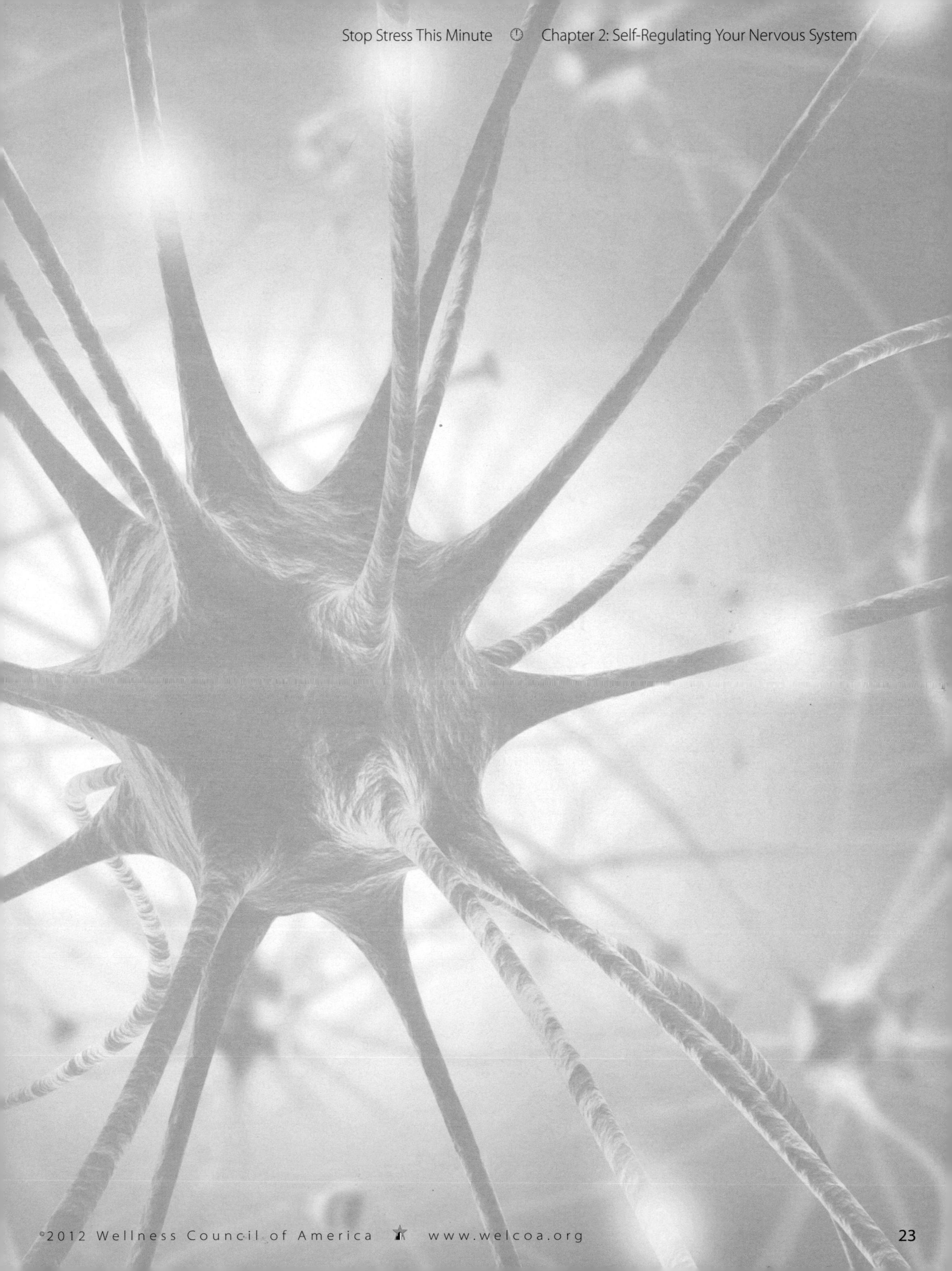

CHAPTER 2

Self-Regulating Your
Nervous System

So what did the Harvard professor, Dr. Herbert Benson, discover back in the sixties when he hooked up those meditators to the biofeedback equipment in his lab? He found that, indeed, they could self-regulate their nervous systems with meditation. They could lower heart rate, breathing rate and metabolism with nothing more than their thoughts. And with further research, he identified other methods that anyone could use to activate what he called "The Relaxation Response," (which is the polar opposite of the stress response.)

In this chapter, we'll demonstrate some of those methods and teach you exactly how to self-regulate your nervous system—in just minutes—using the following ten techniques:

❶ Breathe
❷ Relax
❸ Take Inventory
❹ Stretch
❺ Listen

❻ Focus
❼ Meditate
❽ Visualize
❾ Deep Relaxation
❿ Vigorous Exercise

Before beginning this series of short exercises, take a moment to determine your stress number.

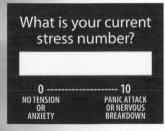

What is your current stress number?

0 ---------------- 10
NO TENSION OR ANXIETY   PANIC ATTACK OR NERVOUS BREAKDOWN

You may also wish to make a note of your stress number before and after each exercise, to see how these ten relaxation techniques compare.

> "It's called the autonomic nervous system (or ANS for short) because it's supposed to work on auto-pilot, without any conscious control by you. Up until the 1960s, most Western scientist believed you couldn't self-regulate your autonomic nervous system."

❶ Breathe

Breathing is one of the few functions of the body that's controlled by the autonomic nervous system (ANS)—and that can also be self-governed. In other words, we can control our breathing whenever we want to—or just let it run on autopilot, as we do most of the time. Generally, the average adult breathes about 12-14 times a minute. In a 24-hour period, that amounts to well over 15,000 breaths a day.

Perhaps as the result of a lifetime of stress, adults learn to breathe shallowly, into the upper part of the lungs. (Watch a baby breathe. They breathe abdominally. Their bellies rise and fall with each breath.) The way adults breathe is known as chest-breathing. There isn't much air exchanged (about a half pint) when we breathe this way, leaving stale air hanging out in the lower lobes of the lungs. If we want to lower our stress number and keep it low, we must remind ourselves to use a breathing technique whenever we feel stressed.

Breathing deeply in the following way also brings in about a gallon of air per breath and is vital to the optimal functioning of the brain. The brain consumes energy at a much higher rate than the rest of the body. And a healthy supply of oxygen supports this high energy consumption.

This simple breathing exercise can help you fall asleep, deal with a stressful encounter while it's happening or even release anger without losing your temper. No matter how you use it, you will be lowering your stress number and thus self-regulating your own nervous system the minute you begin to focus on your breath instead of on your problems.

ABDOMINAL BREATHING EXERCISE

Place your hand over your belly. Take a deep breath in. You can feel your hand rise just slightly on the in-breath. And most likely, you'll feel your hand fall even more on the out-breath. Just focus on your breath and feel your hand rise and fall with each inhalation and exhalation. See if you can make your exhalation last a few seconds longer than your inhalation. Take 3-5 deep breaths in this way or until you feel relaxed.

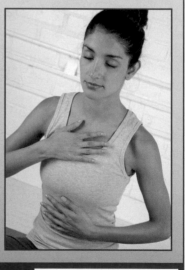

TOTAL TIME:
1 minute

What is your stress number now?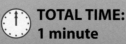

❷ Relax

Dr. Edmund Jacobson published a book in 1934 entitled: *You Must Relax*. In this book, the Harvard-trained MD described a relaxation technique he called Progressive Muscle Relaxation (PMR), which is still in use today. This simple technique was created around the notion that it was easier to teach people how to relax a muscle after deliberately tensing it. That's because people *know* how to make their muscles tense, but they aren't so sure how to relax them. PMR solves this problem by allowing people to first focus on the tension.

The tensing and relaxing cycle of PMR creates a feedback loop that we intuitively understand and can use to manage stress. By tensing a muscle first, we get feedback in terms of palpable feelings and now we know exactly where that muscle is. Most importantly, letting go of the tension in that muscle mimics what we need to do to *begin* relaxing.

In order to facilitate this process, Jacobson instructed his patients to work on different *areas* of the body called muscle groups, tensing and relaxing these areas, one by one. That's why it's sometimes called point by point relaxation. In this *simplified version* of PMR, you'll tense all the muscles of the body at once.

PROGRESSIVE MUSCLE RELAXATION EXERCISE

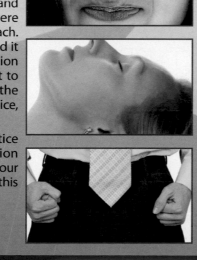

Make a fist with each hand while tensing all the muscles in your body from the top of your head to the tip of your toes. Scrunch your face into the tightest frown you can make, lift your shoulders up to your ears and tighten your belly as if you were about to be poked in the stomach. Take a deep breath in and hold it in while you maintain the tension throughout your body. Count to seven silently and then let all the air and the tension go in one nice, long out-breath.

Breathe in again normally. Notice the growing sense of relaxation and heaviness that remains in your muscles as you do this. Repeat this process three times.

🕐 **TOTAL TIME: 1 minute**

What is your stress number now?

❸ Take Inventory

Some people call this exercise "body scan." It's easy to do, and an effective way to take inventory of the stress that often remains hidden below the surface, trapped in the muscles throughout the body.

It's really quite simple. Sit comfortably in your chair or (if you have more time) lie down on your back and take an imaginary trip through your own body—looking for signs of tension or relaxation—with the goal of increasing the relaxation and reducing the tension. It's a great thing to do right after the previous exercise. (Relaxation is cumulative, just like stress. That's why it's a good idea to keep track of your stress number, as you go, noting it before and after each exercise.)

If you want to get a taste of this body scan technique right now, you can: just move the toes on your left foot. Even if your foot is incarcerated inside a tight shoe, you can still direct your attention there. Close your eyes. Imagine you are traveling right down to the end of your left foot. Can you place your attention there? How do your toes feel? Are they hot? Are they cramped? Are they comfortable? Is there any tension in your toes? Can you relax them just a bit?

BODY SCAN EXERCISE

You'll probably want to do this exercise with your eyes closed. So we'll make the instructions very simple. Starting with your scalp, notice any tension in this area. Breathe in through your nose and let any remaining tension in the area of the scalp float out with your out-breath. Really inhabit each area with the help of your mind's eye. Imagine your breath going right to this area and helping it to relax. Do the same thing in each of the areas listed below. Continue on down through your body stopping at and noticing the muscles around your eyes, your jaw, your neck, your shoulders, your arms, your hands, your belly, your hips, your upper legs, your lower legs, your feet and your toes. After you have scanned each area, breathe in again. Notice any last remaining bit of tension and let it…relax.

🕐 **TOTAL TIME:
1 minute**

What is your stress number now? [   ]

❹ Stretch

Our bodies are a warehouse for tension. Every episode of fight or flight generates muscle tension that tends to sit in our bodies like a tightly wound spring. Eventually, this stored-up tension can lead to problems with back pain, neck pain, headache pain, shoulder spasms and other forms of chronic muscle pain. A great way to unleash this pent up stress is by stretching the muscles out in the following yoga-like postures that you can do while sitting in a chair at home or at work.

STRETCHING EXERCISE

Stretch #1: Spinal Twist

With your feet planted firmly on the floor in front of you and your back straight, reach around to your left and grab the back of the chair with your left hand and the arm of the chair with your right. Move your head gently around to the left also so you are looking at the wall behind you. Breathe in deeply and as you breathe out, pull yourself around to the left and see if you can extend your stretch just a little bit further. Enjoy coming right to the edge of your stretching capability and then let it slowly unwind.

Repeat the above sequence on the right side.

Stretch #2: Shoulder Stretch

Sit a few inches forward on the seat of your chair, feet flat on the floor in front of you. Clasp your hands together behind your back, arch your back and squeeze your shoulder blades together as if you were trying to squeeze a lemon between them. Breathe in and as you breathe out, you have the option to bend forward lifting your clasped hands toward the wall behind you or even higher as you bring your torso down to meet your legs. Hold it there for a few breaths. Come back up and arch your back as you do. Let your hands detach and enjoy the sensations that remain in your body after you let go.

Stretch #3: Overhead Arm Stretch

Hold your hands over your head and stretch. Try to add at least an inch or two to the height of your hands and as you do, you should feel a nice stretch in your upper back. Now drop your shoulders (and arms) down a bit and, take a hold of the left wrist with the right hand and pull your left hand over your head to the right as you bend your torso sideways over to the right, also. You should feel this stretch up the left side of your body and across your back. Repeat on the opposite side. Use your breath to go even deeper into the stretch.

🕐 **TOTAL TIME:**
2 minutes

What is your stress number now?

> "Tension is part and parcel of what we call the mind. Tension does not exist by itself, but is reflexively integrated into the total organism."
>
> —Dr. Edmund Jacobson
> *You Must Relax* (1934)

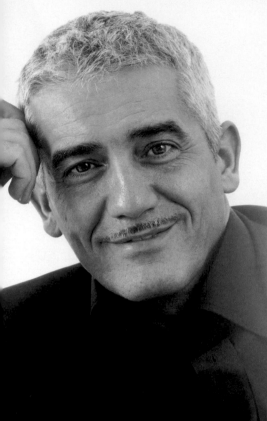

❺ Listen

Years ago, I attended a seminar where Dr. James Lynch of the University of Maryland was demonstrating his research on how blood pressure varies depending on whether we are talking or listening. At this seminar, he asked for volunteers to come up from the audience. He hooked them up to a biofeedback device, and sure enough, when they talked, you could see their blood pressure go up, and when they were listening, you could see it drop.

More recent research shows that when you really connect with a person, your brain will release feel-good chemicals like dopamine and serotonin, making your interaction with that person a potentially healing encounter. Psychologists call this phenomenon: *attunement*. So, listening intently not only lowers your blood pressure and releases feel-good chemicals in the brain, it also promotes better relationships and a sense of being heard and appreciated. So listen more, it's good for your relationships and it's good for your health.

Here's a simple exercise for enhancing your listening skills.

LISTENING EXERCISE

Resist the urge to interrupt. Refer to people by name and look them in the eyes. Ask more questions and really listen to the answers. Don't spend your listening time thinking of what you are going to say next and don't speak until you are SURE the other person is done. Wait a second or two before you begin. Notice the sensations in your brain when you do this.

TOTAL TIME:
2–5 minutes

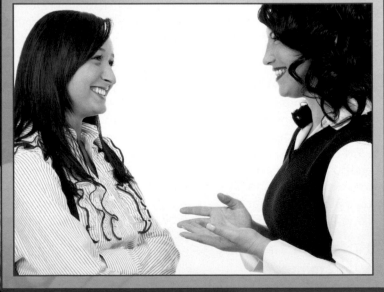

What is your stress number now?

www.welcoa.org   ©2012 Wellness Council of America

❻ Focus

In the last century, people sat at attention for hours listening to long debates and long sermons. Nowadays, most experts believe that "sustained attention" can only be maintained for about 20 minutes. As our daily habits of being attentive expand to include activities such as browsing the Internet, texting, playing video games and viewing short you-tube videos, our attention span is likely to become even shorter. According to the BBC, "most Internet surfers spend less than 60 seconds at the average website."

We pay a price for this lack of focus. When your mind is constantly bouncing around from one thing to another, you'll tend to feel low-level anxiety all the time. That's when your stress number is a 2 or a 3—and you mistakenly assume this slightly anxious state to be your resting state, or zero.

So what can you do to learn how to be more focused and lower your set point back to zero? You need to focus. Why don't you try one of these two exercises right now?

FOCUSING EXERCISES

1. Focus on a spot on the wall with your eyes half shut. It should be a non-descript spot (not a clock ticking or a window looking out on a busy street, or a picture you will be tempted to "think" about.) Just look at this spot for three minutes.

2. Focus on your own breathing. Don't try to change it in any way. Carefully notice every in-breath; every out-breath; and notice the gap between each out-breath and the next in-breath. You may wish to close your eyes while doing this for three minutes.

TOTAL TIME: 3 minutes

What is your stress number now?

Remember when you do either of these two exercises, your mind will wander. That's OK. This happens to EVERYONE. Don't let it bother you. Just keep bringing it back to the point of focus—even if you have to do this 100 times in three minutes.

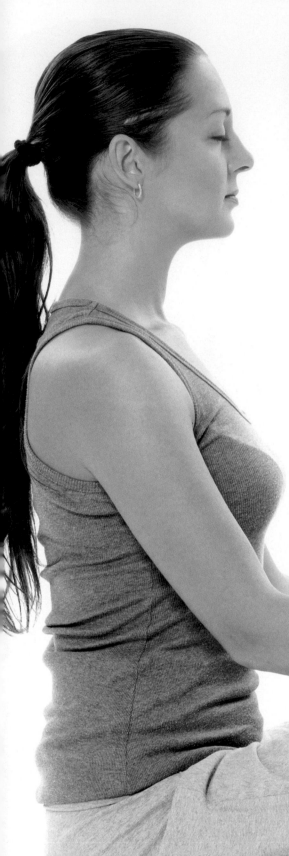

❼ Meditate

There seems to be something about meditation that turns a lot of people off. Maybe it's because in pictures you always see people sitting cross-legged on the floor, (you can sit up in a chair), or maybe it's because people think you need a secret "mantra," (almost any relaxing word or phrase will do), or maybe it's because people wonder how you can possibly benefit from sitting still for long periods of time where you are essentially doing nothing, (you can start with just five minutes a day—and learning how to concentrate is NOT doing nothing.) Despite these misconceptions, the research on meditation is crystal clear and the benefits to be derived from this ancient practice are many.

Psychologists describe these benefits as "state and trait effects." State effects refer to pleasant feelings of relaxation that occur while you meditate. Trait effects refer to the long term changes that occur in the brain as the result of meditating. Regular meditators have been reporting changes like improved mood, feeling more relaxed, increased patience with people and things, better ability to focus, more control over their emotions and increased productivity—for as long as meditation has been in practice.

But now, with the advent of brain imaging equipment, we can actually map these trait effects to see how the brain changes as a person's meditation practice deepens. Over time, the areas of the brain that keep stress under control get stronger and slightly bigger (more neural pathways) and the areas of the brain that tend to initiate stress get weaker and slightly smaller (less neural pathways.)

In his book, *The Relaxation Response*, Dr. Herbert Benson condensed the teaching of meditation into a few very simple steps. You can practice this exercise to help you reduce your stress almost immediately.

MEDITATION EXERCISE

Before you begin meditating, you will need:

1. A quiet space where you won't be disturbed.
2. A comfortable position. (This could be sitting in a chair with both feet flat on the floor and with your back straight.)
3. A word or phrase to help you stay focused.*
4. A passive attitude.

Choose a word or phrase to repeat silently to yourself, over and over. Some good candidates are: ONE, PEACE, RELAX, or I AM FEELING MORE AND MORE RELAXED. You may wish to close your eyes while doing this.

🕐 **TOTAL TIME:**
5 minutes

What is your stress number now?

Sometimes the hardest part of meditating is maintaining a passive attitude. A lot of Type-A personalities have trouble meditating because they push too hard and attempt to force themselves into a meditative state. This just won't work. You have to just relax and let it happen.

Also, don't be too concerned by the fact that your mind wanders to and fro while you meditate. Just keep bringing it back to your word or phrase and eventually you will get the hang of it. Your word or phrase will become "an operant conditioner," just like the bell that caused Pavlov's dogs to salivate. With repeated practice, you'll come to associate this word or phrase with the feeling of relaxation (just like Pavlov's dogs associated the sound of the bell with the taste of food.) When that starts to happen, your meditation will become easier and easier.

Begin with a short meditation practice of only five minutes, and if it's convenient, do it first thing in the morning. After this short practice becomes a habit, you may want to add more minutes over time. Most people eventually end up meditating for longer periods, but don't let that stop you from meditating for just five minutes at the beginning. You have to start somewhere and this is a great place to begin.

> "Our minds want to be challenged and crave focus. Concentrating on something for longer periods of time will improve our ability to focus."

STRESS SYMPTOMS

- Headaches
- Neck aches
- Heartburn
- Stomach pain
- Dry mouth
- Cold hands
- Irritability
- Anxiety
- Negative attitude
- Sleeplessness
- Crying spells
- Difficulty making decisions
- Lethargy
- Low mood
- Difficulty concentrating
- Disorganization
- Cynicism
- Elevated blood pressure
- Low libido
- Fidgeting or feet tapping
- Arguing more
- Apathy
- Accident prone
- Rashes or hives
- Teeth-grinding
- Loss of appetite
- Emotional eating (eating to calm yourself)
- Increased smoking, alcohol or drug use
- Excessive gambling
- Impulse buying
- Loneliness
- Not caring about appearance

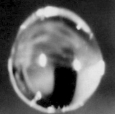

❽ Visualize

Visualization, also known as guided imagery, can be as simple as a golfer imagining what the perfect drive might look like and then rehearsing it in his or her head, or as complicated as a breast cancer patient imagining her immune-system firing up to aid a course of chemotherapy. Guided imagery has been used successfully to help professional athletes play better—and to help average people overcome all sorts of health problems from cancer to chronic pain.

According to Belleruth Naparstek, an author and expert on the subject, "just ten minutes of guided imagery a day can reduce blood pressure, lower cholesterol, and heighten short term immune cell activity. It lessens headaches and pain, reduces anxiety, and even reduces the adverse effects of chemotherapy."

Your body can't tell the difference between when you are imagining something and when you are actually doing it. If you vividly imagine climbing up a rock ledge, your body will release some of the same stress chemicals it would if you were actually climbing that cliff. So, in order to use visualization to lower your stress, you'll want to IMAGINE something VERY relaxing. Since everyone experiences stress and relaxing events differently, you will need to customize this exercise to your own needs. (Some people find beaches relaxing, other people don't.)

> "Just ten minutes of guided imagery a day can reduce blood pressure, lower cholesterol, and heighten short term immune cell activity. It lessens headaches and pain, reduces anxiety, and even reduces the adverse effects of chemotherapy."
>
> —Belleruth Naparstek

Read the directions below before starting this exercise, and customize it to suit your needs. Just imagine yourself relaxing deeply in whatever scene you choose.

VISUALIZATION EXERCISE

A lot of people need help visualizing, so if you are one of those, keep a picture of your favorite vacation spot on your desk or workstation. (Or use the picture you see here.) In any case, lock this image into your mind. It could be a beach or on a dock by a lake, or in the mountains or walking through your favorite park.

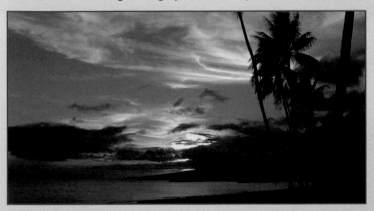

Close your eyes now, and put yourself in your favorite relaxing spot. This is your private place and no one will disturb you here. Breathe in deeply. If you're on a beach or in the country, it may help to imagine the sounds of the waves lapping up on the shore, the birds crying out in the distance and/or the crickets humming in background.

There's a gentle breeze blowing and the air is the perfect temperature. You can feel the warm sun on your face. You notice the leaves swaying in the breeze and you feel just a hint of coolness across your forehead. Breathing in again, feel yourself relax into the cozy comfort of your protected place.

For the next few minutes, you're free to explore this special place. Bask in the warm sun, or take an imaginary stroll, or feel the wind in your face as you float along. Really inhabit this place in your mind, knowing that for the time being, you are completely safe from anything that could possibly harm you or bother you.

When you feel totally at ease, notice your breathing. How does it feel? Notice the air around your skin. How does that feel? Notice sensations inside your body. How does that feel? Focus on the relaxation growing throughout your whole body from your head to your toes. Let it wash over you leaving you feeling deeply, deeply relaxed.

**TOTAL TIME:
5 minutes**

What is your stress number now?

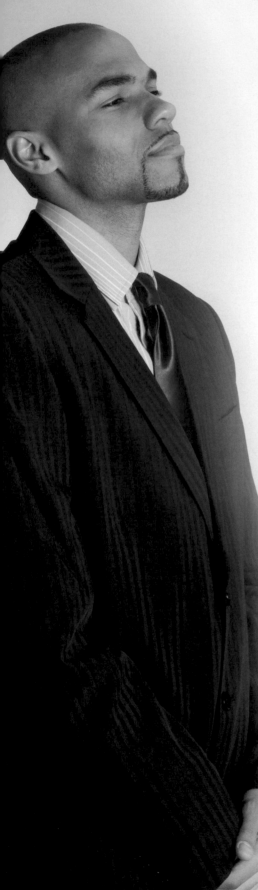

❾ Deep Relaxation

This technique is often called self-hypnosis and is a superb way to relax, deeply. Self-hypnosis is different from regular hypnosis in that you are in total control of your experience. Basically, anytime you are self-regulating your ANS, you are putting yourself into an "altered state of consciousness." This is different from your everyday waking state of consciousness, which is often characterized by low-level anxiety, faster brain waves and a heightened sense of alertness.

When you direct yourself into a deeply relaxed state, your consciousness changes, your brain waves slow down, your breathing rate slows and your heart rate slows down, too. As with many of the previous exercises, you may wish to close your eyes. If so, you'll want to familiarize yourself with the instructions before beginning.

DEEP RELAXATION EXERCISE

You are going to simply count backwards from ten. Each number will take you deeper and deeper into relaxation. Be sure to say each number silently to yourself as you go. Take this very, very slowly.

10. **Breathing in, deeply.**
9. **Getting more and more relaxed.**
8. **Breathing in again, deeply.**
7. **Feeling the relaxation growing throughout the whole body.**
6. **Breathing in through the nose and out through the partially closed mouth.**
5. **Hands are feeling heavy and warm.**
4. **Arms are feeling heavy and warm.**
3. **My whole body is feeling heavy and warm.**
2. **Breathing in again, deeply.**
1. **I am now deeply, deeply relaxed.**

You can repeat this countdown as often you like.

🕐 **TOTAL TIME: 2 minutes**

What is your stress number now?

> "When you direct yourself into a deeply relaxed state, your consciousness changes, your brain waves slow down, your breathing rate slows and your heart rate slows down, too."

⑩ Vigorous Exercise

If you could put all the benefits of exercise into the form of a pill, everyone would take it. Besides lowering the risk of diabetes, high blood pressure and heart disease, regular exercise helps you lower stress. According to John Ratey MD, author of the book, *Spark*, exercise "raises the fight or flight threshold," (so you are less likely to be startled by loud noises, lose your temper, or behave in ways you'll later regret.) You're quite simply, more resilient to stress. According to Ratey, "on a mechanical level, exercise relaxes the resting tension of muscle spindles, which breaks the stress-feedback loop to the brain. If the body isn't stressed, the brain figures maybe it can relax too."

When I was considering a form of vigorous exercise for reducing stress, I wasn't sure I could come up with something that would only take a couple of minutes. I tried climbing stairs and, for me, that didn't work, although it might for you (so that's included below.) Then I had a little brainstorm. What about jumping rope? I hadn't tried it in years, but a trainer had once told me that it was UBER AEROBIC! So, I found a jump rope at the YMCA where I work out every day, and somehow, after two or three false starts I got the hang of it. I noticed as I watched the clock that I was doing about one jump per second and it seemed like a fairly doable pace (since I'm pretty much a total novice at it.) So when I counted to 60 twice, I had jump-roped for about two minutes. I was exhausted! I normally exercise vigorously for a half an hour, five days a week, so I couldn't believe how quickly this got my heart pumping.

VIGOROUS EXERCISE

If you want to get your heart pumping and use the benefits of exercise to reduce stress almost immediately, try one of the vigorous activities listed here (or create one of your own.)

Please Note: Before beginning ANY exercise program, you should consult your doctor. These 2-minute exercises are intense and may surprise you, especially if you haven't exercised lately.

- ⏱ Vigorous Exercise Option #1: Jump Rope
- ⏱ Vigorous Exercise Option #2: Climb Stairs

🕐 **TOTAL TIME:
2 minutes**

What is your stress number now?* [   ]

Allow a cool down period of a few minutes before taking your stress number.

Self-Regulation In Summary

Remember, not all techniques work for all people. That's why we covered ten different techniques in this chapter, with many more techniques yet to come in later chapters. Even if only ONE of these stress-reduction techniques proves useful to you and you begin to practice it on a regular basis, the net effect could be life-changing. Don't underestimate the power that one small change can bring about.

Also remember how the stress number system works. Stress is often cumulative, so you don't want to let it build, one stressful event after another, without doing something to control it or counteract it. In the first chapter, you learned how your levels of stress hormones rise and fall throughout the day, while building on the stress hormone levels that immediately preceded them. So, if you're ignoring your rising levels of stress, eventually you will pay a price in terms of your peace of mind, your personal welfare, your health and how well you get along with others.

As you monitor your stress throughout the day with the stress number system, a good tip is to never let your stress level get above a 5 without doing something to change directions. If you're at work, breathe—if you're at home, exercise—or focus or relax. If none of those options are suitable, simply do something a little differently—change desks, work on a different task, call a customer or client that you actually LIKE, or just do whatever you have to do to nudge that number back down in the other direction.

In the next two chapters we'll discuss how your mind creates stress and what you can do to stop it. ☉

> "As you monitor your stress throughout the day with the stress number system, a good tip is to never let your stress level get above a 5 without doing something to change directions."

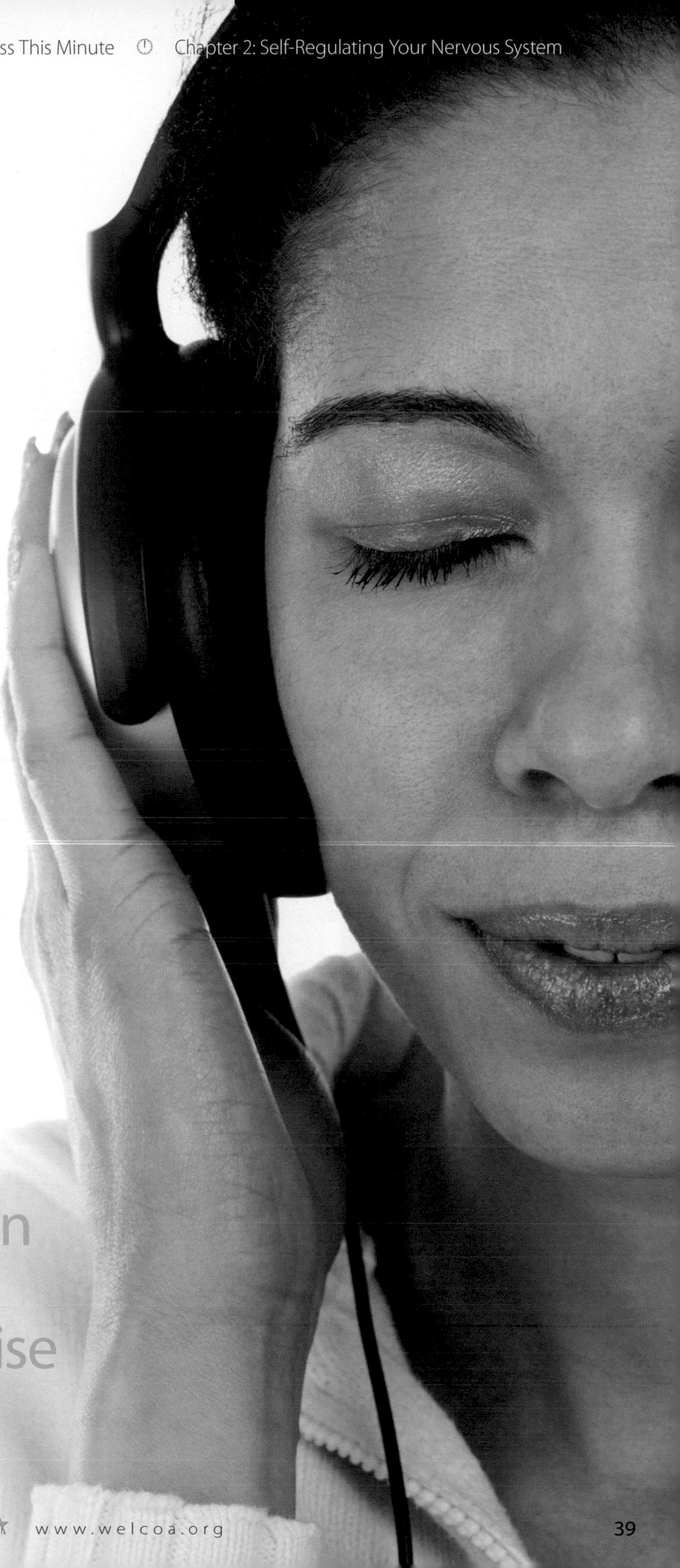

❶ Breathe

❷ Relax

❸ Take Inventory

❹ Stretch

❺ Listen

❻ Focus

❼ Meditate

❽ Visualize

❾ Deep Relaxation

❿ Vigorous Exercise

CHAPTER 3

What Is The #1 Source Of Stress?

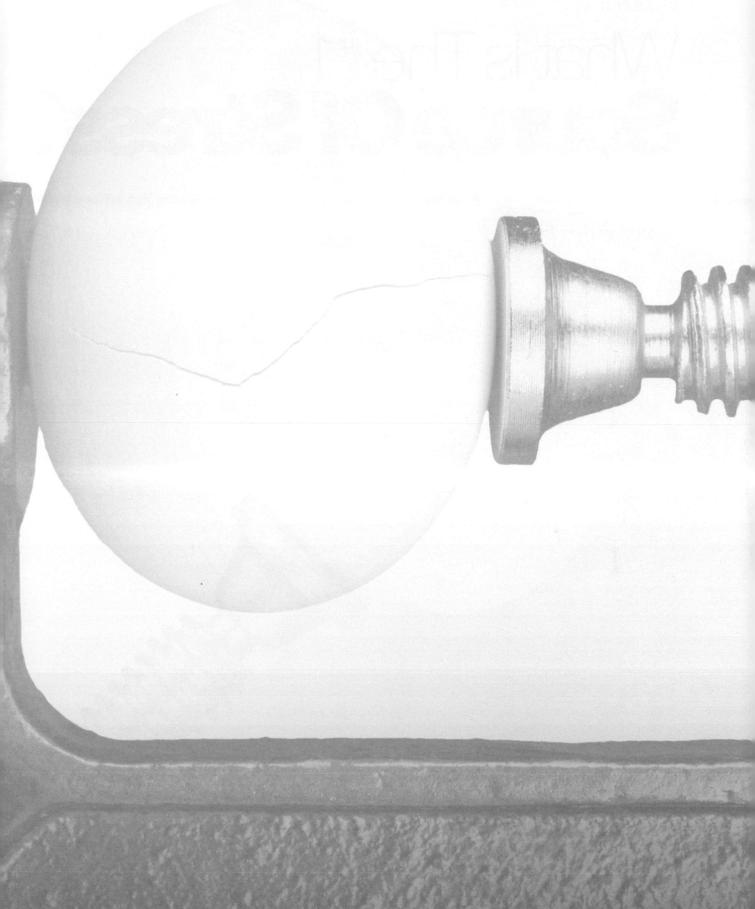

CHAPTER 3

What Is The #1
Source Of Stress?

Have you ever wondered what the number one source of stress in your life is? According the American Psychological Association, the top two sources of stress are job stress and financial pressure. But what if *we* said the number one source of stress in your life is *you*?

Up until this very moment you've been *programmed* to believe that your stress is the result of outside factors you can't control. You get a flat tire and you feel stressed. Someone cuts ahead of you in line and you feel stressed. Your spouse blames you for something you didn't do and you feel stressed. Your boss criticizes your work unfairly and you feel stressed. Since you can't control what happens to you, how can you possibly control your stress? It's just a simple cause and effect relationship: a stressful event happens and you feel stressed, right?

Wrong. (Actually this is the second stress management myth.)

Stress Management Myth #2

Stress is not JUST the result of what happens to you—because there's one major piece missing from this deduction. Can you guess what it is?

It's you, or more accurately, your thinking. In other words, how you think about or interpret what happens to you. And when you factor in your interpretation, you quickly see that stress IS the result of a cause and effect relationship, but the relationship ISN'T so simple. It's more complicated.

The *actual way* a stressful event unfolds is what we call the *sequence of stress*. Here's how it works.

Let's say you walk out to your car in the morning and discover that you have a flat tire. You're on your way to work and you're in a hurry. The sequence of stress is as follows: First comes **the event** (the flat tire); next come **your thoughts and beliefs** about that event; and finally, **your reaction**.

Now, despite what you might think, your reaction isn't automatically going to be stressful. *It depends on what your thoughts and beliefs are about the flat tire.*

If, after seeing your tire you have thoughts like: *This flat tire is going to take forever to fix. It's the worst possible thing that could have happened to me at the worst possible moment. Now I'll never get to work on time*—of course you are going to feel stressed!

> "When you blame outside events and circumstances for your stress such as a flat tire... you're only considering half of the story."

Life's Neutral Events

Now here's one of the most difficult points to understand about stress: Most events are neutral—but we attach meaning to them with our thoughts and beliefs. Take snow for example. Kids love it, adults generally hate it. What happens between childhood and adulthood? We attach different meanings to it. When we're kids snow represents fun and frolic and a day off from school. When we're adults, it usually means more work, difficulty driving, traffic jams and childcare.

The snow doesn't change. It's neutral. Our thoughts and beliefs about the snow changes and thus our reaction to it changes as well. Even an event as unquestionably significant as death can be seen as a blessing (or a curse) depending upon the thoughts and beliefs of the person who's thinking them.

So, it's only when a neutral event is combined with your *negative* thoughts and beliefs that *it adds up to stress*.

When you blame outside events and circumstances for your stress such as a flat tire, someone cutting ahead of you in line, an argument with your spouse or boss, etc., you're only considering half of the story. When it comes to stress, your thinking—your thoughts and beliefs—is actually a MAJOR source of that stress. Possibly, the biggest source of stress—and there are some *cognitive* psychologists who might say the ONLY source.

Dr. Albert Ellis, who wrote the book *How To Stubbornly Refuse To Make Yourself Miserable About Anything—Yes Anything*, is generally acknowledged as THE FIRST cognitive psychologist. (Cognitive refers to thinking.) In his books, Dr. Ellis tells the stories of patients whose thinking caused them to experience stress. For example, if a patient was complaining about her husband who was "always tracking mud in the house," Ellis would zero in on the patient's thinking:

"Did your husband track mud in the house today?"

"No," the patient would reply.

"Did he track mud in the house yesterday?"

"No."

"When was the last time your husband tracked mud in the house?"

"About a week ago."

Rational Emotive Behavioral Therapy (REBT) And Cognitive Behavioral Therapy (CBT)

It was the year 1955. A light bulb went off in Ellis's head. He realized something that would eventually change the way psychologists would practice their art around the world: EVERYONE occasionally thinks *irrationally*. And, this irrational thinking causes them to experience a significant amount of *unnecessary* pain. What's even more surprising, Ellis discovered, is *that people seldom realize that they think this way*. Ellis concluded that if he could make people aware of how to change their thinking, they could "fix their own problems" much more quickly than they could through traditional psychoanalysis. He then started a new form of therapy that was based on these ideas.

Ellis called his new form of therapy Rational Emotive Behavioral Therapy or REBT for short. (Aaron Beck MD, started writing about this same subject a few years after Ellis. Even though Ellis came first, the world adopted Beck's name—Cognitive Behavioral Therapy or CBT—for this new therapy focused on a patient's thinking.) Ellis and Beck's work would ultimately streamline the course of treatment for a typical patient from a process that often took years to something that could be accomplished in a matter of a few one-hour sessions. This also revolutionized the whole field of psychology because it was found that even "healthy people" could benefit from these cognitive techniques as well.

If you've ever heard the words "awfulizing" or "catastrophizing," or the expression "stop shoulding on yourself," (such as *I should have made my bed; I should have done the laundry; I should have worn a better outfit*), these are words and phrases that Dr. Ellis coined to help his patients understand how their thoughts and beliefs affected their emotions and behaviors.

Sixty years after Ellis and Beck first started writing about this subject, we have numerous medical studies that prove the effectiveness of CBT as a form of therapy. For example, studies show that 13 weeks of cognitive therapy is as effective as anti-depressants in relieving depression.

Activating + Belief = Consequence

So, let's go back to the example of the flat tire and you will understand how this approach can help you to relieve stress. The thoughts and beliefs were: *This flat tire is going to take forever to fix. It's the worst possible thing that could have happened at the worst possible time. Now I'll never get to work on time.*

Basically, because this event isn't happening now, it's easy to see that these remarks are *irrational* and *overly exaggerated*. But if it were happening to you right now, you might be thinking these exact same thoughts and not even realize it. This internal dialogue is what psychologists call "negative self-talk."

Maybe you've heard yourself say things like: *"This traffic jam is taking forever. I've got the world's worst boss. This task is impossible. I'll never finish this assignment. Why does this stuff always happen to me? My spouse is always nagging me. My co-worker is never on time for anything. This car is always breaking down. I can't stand it when that happens."*

Our minds constantly run an inner dialogue about everything we do, almost like the play-by-play commentator at a sporting event. We can actually observe (and listen to) this negative self-talk anytime we want, but for some reason, perhaps because it's so pervasive, we usually don't. So, as a result, it continues on just below our radar without us being fully conscious of it. Thus, events taking place all around us are experienced—without us realizing—through our "filter" of negative thinking. This subconscious filter of play-by-play commentary is often overly negative, muddled and exaggerated.

> "Our minds constantly run an inner dialogue about everything thing we do, almost like the play-by-play commentator at a sporting event."

At this point you may be shaking your head and saying, "So what? What's the big deal if my thinking is a little negative? What's the harm in that?"

Actually there's a lot of harm in it. As you learned from the opening examples, stress is the result of events that happen to us—plus our thinking about those events. So, if your thinking is overly negative and irrational, you are going experience a lot more stress.

Luckily, Albert Ellis came up with a simple equation to help us sort this all out, and it's as easy to remember as **ABC**. The **A**ctivating event plus your **B**elief equals the **C**onsequence. **A + B = C**.

In the opening example, the flat tire is the **A**ctivating event, or **A**. One of the **B**eliefs, or **B**, is that this flat tire *is going to take forever to fix*. The **C**onsequence, or **C**, is the stress one feels inside as the result of **A + B**. In this case, if the flat tire had happened to you, you might have felt frustrated or upset. That's why allowing this negative self-talk to go on unnoticed and uncorrected is going to lead to a lot of unnecessary stress.

We know from the stress number system that when you think irrationally, you are dialing up your stress number. When you think rationally, you are dialing it down. We also know that when you dial it up, you are more likely to add on additional layers of irrationality like *"Why do these things always happen to me? This is the worst possible thing that could happen at the worst possible moment. Now I'll never get to work on time."*

Ellis liked to say that we need to look out for the words "always" and "never" in our thinking. They are like red flags, he would say, letting us know that our thinking is probably irrational or exaggerated. People are complex and seldom do we always (or never) do things one way or another. Usually it's somewhere in between. But our mind likes to paint our interpretations in shades of black or white. Beck called this *all or nothing* thinking.

Ellis and Beck started a revolution by pointing out that a lot of thinking tends to be irrational and overly negative. People often (with good reason) confuse the cognitive approach to managing stress with positive thinking, but it's NOT the same.

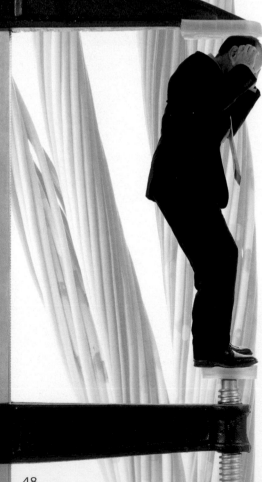

We have now shattered two myths about stress management. Can you remember the second one? If so, write it down.

....

....

....

....

....

Hint: Stressful events always cause us to feel stressed. True or false?

The cognitive approach is about recognizing that much of our thinking is OVERLY negative and exaggerated: *I'll never amount to anything. Life is so unfair. This task is impossible. My coworker is of absolutely no use at all. Meetings are a complete waste of my time I'm a terrible parent. I'm no good at anything.*

All Beck and Ellis want us to do is:

1. Become aware of our overly negative thinking and realize that it goes on all the time.

2. Try to neutralize it—But not necessarily make it positive. Simply, keep our thinking from being overly negative.

When a flat tire happens on the highway, it's not a JOYFUL event. No one is saying it is. Basically, it's a nuisance, but it's NOT the end of the world either. It's not a catastrophe. And when we interpret it OVERLY negatively, which we often do, it adds immeasurably to our stress.

One final thought about this thinking person's approach to managing stress, or what some psychologists call cognitive restructuring: One might be tempted to say that lowering your stress is easy as changing your thinking. While this statement is basically true, changing your thinking ISN'T always easy—especially, as it turns out, because thoughts and beliefs are often hard-wired.

What does that mean, hard-wired? With the flat tire example, you can hear your own irrational thoughts, so these beliefs are easier to dispute. They're not hard-wired.

With hard-wired beliefs, you often don't hear any self-talk. Your reaction just happens. A lifetime of behavioral conditioning has reduced you to certain predictable knee-jerk responses: You may hate traffic jams, or spiders or noisy neighbors or dogs because one of your parents hated these same things and taught YOU to hate them too.

When your beliefs are hard-wired, it seems like A = C and there is no B in the equation at all. And this is the way the whole world thinks! On some level you know darned well how you are going to react before that button is even pushed! But you never take the time to think about whether you could change your reaction, or disable that hard-wired belief.

If you're stuck in this way, you can learn to get unstuck and you can learn to control your reaction—even under challenging circumstances—with repeated practice.

You do this by FIRST, becoming aware of what your hot buttons are (make a list), and SECOND, by substituting new thoughts and new beliefs for old outmoded beliefs and the irrational thinking that no longer serves you. Every time you see a hot button about to be pressed, you have to force yourself to choose how you're going to react, to think in new ways. (Make a second list of new substitute thoughts and behaviors to draw from.)

As Stephen Covey put it in his book, *The Eighth Habit*, all your opportunity for personal growth lies in the small space between stimulus and response. (Between cause and effect, or between A and C.) In the next chapter, we're going to show you how to inhabit that small space and by so doing, change your whole world. ⊙

MAKE A LIST OF YOUR TOP FIVE HOT BUTTONS

Example of a hot button: *I get really defensive (and sometimes angry) when people criticize my work.*

Usual results of hard-wired reaction: *I make it difficult for people to communicate with me when they are not happy with my work.*

New thoughts and/or behavior: *When people criticize my work, I'll consciously take a deep breath in. Then I will be able to react calmly.*

Top five hot buttons:

❶
❷
❸
❹
❺

What usually happens when a hot button gets pressed?

❶
❷
❸
❹
❺

New thoughts and behaviors:

❶
❷
❸
❹
❺

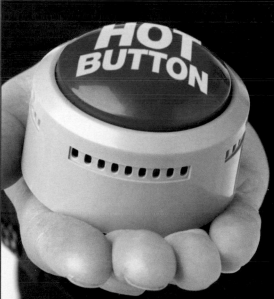

CHAPTER 4

I Think Therefore
I'm Stressed

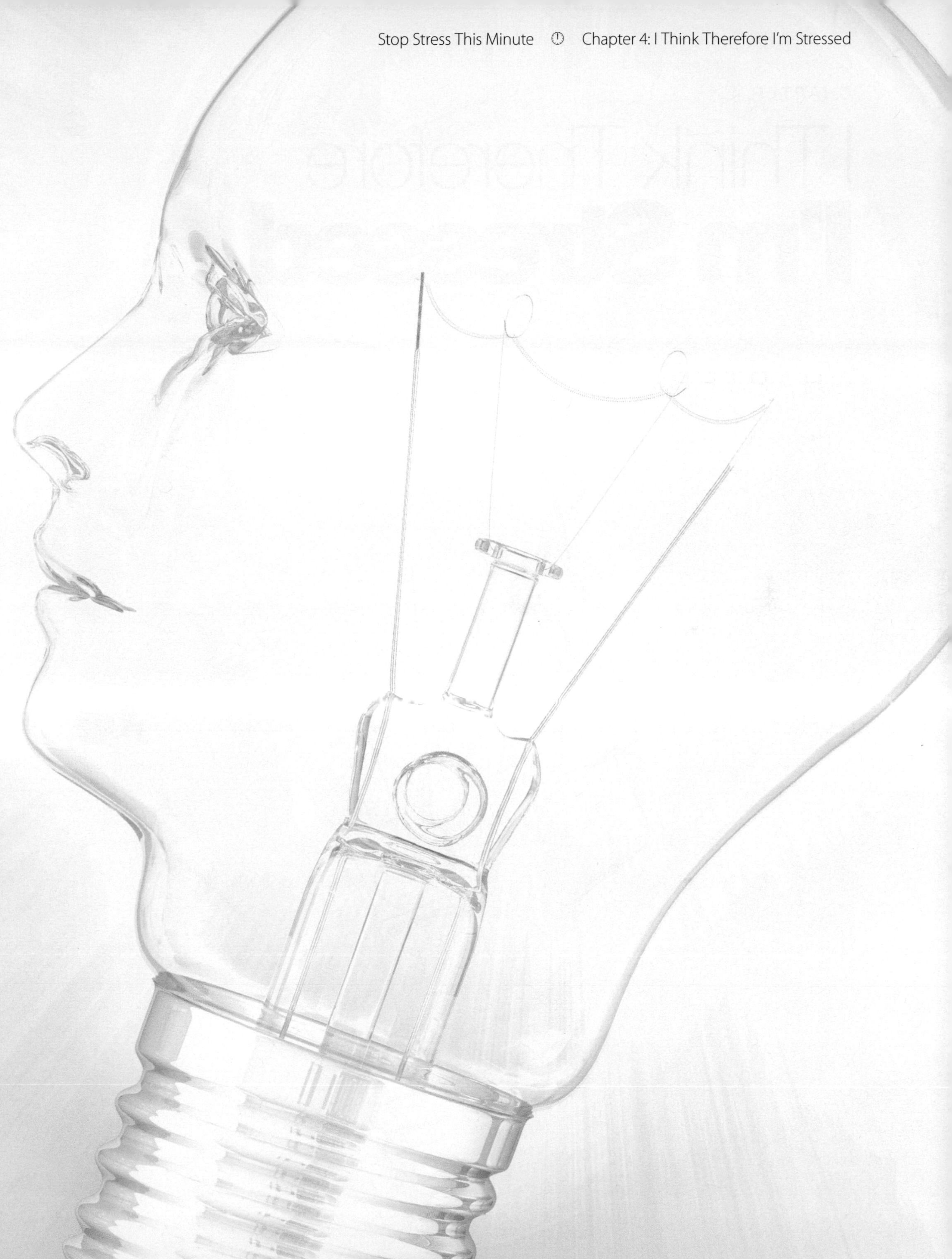

CHAPTER 4

I Think Therefore
I'm Stressed

The great thing about cognitive techniques for managing stress is that they take absolutely NO time at all. Once you've read the previous chapter and memorized the five cognitive, stress-management techniques you'll learn in this chapter—that's it—you're pretty much done. You don't have to spend time at the gym practicing them. You don't have to sit in a quiet room and meditate on them. You don't have to visualize yourself saying them. You don't even have to hold hands with the person next to you and sing Kumbaya!

The following five techniques will not only help you stop stress this minute, but they will help you stop it this *second*. You just have to believe in them and keep invoking these techniques at every opportunity.

In a series of front page articles about stress in the workplace, *The New York Times* wrote: *"The one workplace stress-reduction technique that seems to out-perform all others is cognitive restructuring."*

Changing your thinking, (which is exactly what cognitive restructuring means), requires a commitment to transformation that many people *are not prepared to make*. That's because altering your thinking isn't easy. Henry Ford summed this up beautifully when he said: "Whether you think you can or you think you can't; *either way you're right.*"

The good news is you can change your thinking and those deeply ingrained thinking *patterns*. Daniel Siegel MD, a psychiatrist and professor at UCLA, writes about neuroplasticity and the brain in his book, *Mindsight*. Neuroplasticity is the new buzz word in brain science and it simply refers to the ability of the brain to change and grow. Scientists used to think the brain stopped changing and growing in childhood, but now, with the research done by Siegel and others, we know our bodies manufacture thousands of new neurons *every day*. The brain changes constantly throughout our lifetimes in response to experience. In his book, Dr. Siegel writes about his patients—some of whom are in their nineties—and their ability to rewire their own brains to make permanent cognitive and behavioral changes that transform their whole lives.

This chapter is going to teach you five cognitive, stress-management techniques that will assist you in reshaping and rewiring your own brain. These five techniques will help you change your habits, your behaviors and the way you *think* about stressful problems—because in many cases, the only thing standing between you and your new behaviors is A SINGLE THOUGHT.

> "Changing your thinking, (which is exactly what cognitive restructuring means), requires a commitment to transformation that many people are not prepared to make. That's because altering your thinking isn't easy."

❶ D Stands For Dispute

After Dr. Albert Ellis created his now famous A + B = C equation, he realized there was an important piece missing. The equation doesn't tell you how to *change* your thinking at B. So that's when he came up with the letter D, for Dispute.

Ellis often said: "Man is the only animal on the planet that can think about his thinking." So, as the result of this amazing ability we are able to *observe* when our thinking is irrational, muddled, or overly negative—and once we do—we are also able to *dispute* this irrational thinking. For example, when you hear yourself say: *"I've got the world's worst boss,"* you can immediately start the dispute process with thoughts like: *"How could I possibly even know this without comparing him or her to all the other bosses in the world?"*

Sometimes our irrational thinking is just ridiculous and we need to recognize this. One of Ellis' favorite irrational statements to dispute was "I can't stand it when (that) happens." (Whatever that might be.) He realized it's an irrational statement because *as soon as hear yourself say it, you have already withstood whatever it is.* So you obviously *can* stand it!

Of course you don't have the world's worst boss, and a traffic jam couldn't possibly take forever, and the endless meetings ALL come to an end. So on the surface, our negative thinking is often just flat-out wrong. And that's the first level of irrationality we need to dispute. But we can learn to dispute these internal thoughts on a deeper level too.

To enhance your dispute, think of some real-life examples of times that refute your irrational self-talk: *My boss did let me go home early last week, when I wasn't feeling well. When I got stuck in traffic yesterday it only took five minutes for the traffic to clear. Last week's staff meeting wasn't long at all.* You are not trying to sugar coat ANYTHING, only sort out what's true and what's not, and the thinking that's overly negative. Remember you are the one who suffers for your irrational thinking so there's motivation for sorting this out. Since you are the one who suffers, you are the one who needs to dispute these thoughts and beliefs at every opportunity.

www.welcoa.org ★

❷ Stop Passing Judgment

Believe it or not, passing judgment is a major source of stress. We all have judgments about everything, all the time. For example, that *people shouldn't talk in movie theatres, people shouldn't cut in line, people shouldn't take advantage of me,* and *people should always be considerate.* We also have judgments about ourselves: *I must never embarrass myself in public, I must always appear successful.* (Beck called these self-statements *unwritten rules*.)

We have judgments about how long we should wait in line at the bank and we even have judgments about what the appropriate colors are for our neighbor's house. *(A purple house? That's ghastly!)* And let's not forget our children. *They should always be polite. They should get along with each other and they should never talk back to their parents.*

I realized how rampant my own judging had become—and how much stress it was causing me—when I started talking about crabgrass with my 21-year-old son.

"Why do you care so much about crabgrass, Dad?"

"Can't you see how *ugly* it is?" I asked him.

"Quite frankly Dad, I can't. Now tell me, which is the crabgrass and which is regular grass?"

Right then and there, I realized how much pain this judgment was causing me—and he couldn't even tell the difference between the crabgrass and the regular grass! As an adult, I had learned to dislike crab grass. I would have to TEACH my son to hate it, too. And like most judgments—in the larger scheme of things—it was an incredibly minor issue and yet it was causing me a significant amount of extra work, struggle and stress.

(This is not to say that you shouldn't do something about your crabgrass. But when you do: Realize that you've *learned* to dislike crabgrass and many other things in your life that were once simply neutral and had absolutely no effect on you *whatsoever*.)

> "Remember to ask yourself, every time you hear yourself judging someone or something, who is experiencing the stress as the result of the judgment? Not the person or thing you are judging—it's YOU."

In order to get over this cognitive hurdle of always passing judgment, you must first become aware of just how frequently you are doing it. For most people, it's constant. We judge our spouses, our children our friends, our neighbors and of course total strangers—even the grass! Remember to ask yourself, every time you hear yourself judging someone or something, *who is experiencing the stress as the result of the judgment?* Not the person or thing you are judging—it's YOU.

You can easily prove this to yourself. Have you ever fallen asleep with the TV on or slept through a thunderstorm? Sure, just about everybody has. Well, the next time you are awakened by a racket in the middle of the night, notice whether it's the noise or your JUDGMENT about the PERSON who made the noise that's keeping you awake. After all, if you can fall asleep with the TV blasting, or sleep through a thunderstorm, noise is probably NOT the issue. It's oftentimes your judgment that is causing you to lie awake and *suffer*.

THE FIVE COGNITIVE STRESS-MANAGEMENT TECHNIQUES

1. **D Stands For Dispute**
2. **Stop Passing Judgment**
3. **Only Worry With A Writing Instrument**
4. **Accept What Is And Can't Be Changed**
5. **Keep Your Stress In Perspective**

❸ Only Worry With A Writing Instrument

My mother thoroughly trained me in the fine art of WORRY. Every day she'd comb the local paper for articles about kids who met their untimely demise mostly because they "didn't think."

There were the kids who stuck knives in toasters, there were the kids who took the short-cut home by crossing the railroad tracks. There was the kid who was painting his house and leaned an aluminum ladder against a power line. And there was the poor 10-year-old girl who died of rabies, who wasn't even aware of being bitten by a bat because she had slept right through it.

And the message I took away from all those scary articles was that using a toaster, going anywhere near a train, painting a house, and even SLEEPING could all be FATAL. As a result of this high-level training in all that could possibly go disastrously wrong in life, I used to worry excessively.

It was no small feat to conquer this worry-habit which my dear mother had so carefully instilled in me. Habits usually get cultivated over the course of a lifetime and worriers are in the habit of worrying. But habits are learned and can also be unlearned.

That's why this lesson is to *only worry with a writing instrument.* You can't write while you're doing the dishes, while you're driving, or taking a shower, or lying in a dark bedroom in the middle of the night. So don't worry during those times either. When worries come into your mind, consciously say to yourself: *I'm not going to worry about those things now. I'll worry later when I can do something about them.*

I'm not saying DON'T worry. All I'm saying is don't waste your time worrying when you can't write your problems down, and by so doing, set in motion a process that would eventually solve them. When you write your problems down, they stop swirling around in your head where they can actually make you tense.

So remember, only worry with a writing instrument. Which simply means that yes, it's important to worry when you can truly FOCUS on your worries, write them down, and to the greatest degree possible, reduce the odds of them coming true. But over and above that, you must get OUT of the habit of worrying at ALL other times like the middle of the night, or while you are driving, or doing the dishes. This kind of worry has no value—and contributes a lot of hidden stress.

❹ Accept What Is And Can't Be Changed

When your sixteen year old gets a tattoo or a body-piercing you don't like, how do you accept what is and can't be changed? When you've been told that your job is being cutback, how do you accept what is and can't be changed? When your doctor tells you you've got cancer, how do you accept what is and can't be changed?

When is it EVER better to just accept the way things turn out rather than to ferociously fight to change them back to the way they were? And in the case of cancer, what are you supposed to do, just roll over and die?

But what if you knew, even on your deathbed, that you were only one thought away from inner-peace and serenity? Wouldn't you want to know what that thought, or bit of advice might be?

Well here it is: you have an opportunity at any given moment of being happy or being upset. Whether it's accepting yourself, or accepting others, or simply accepting a situation that can't be changed, oftentimes the doorway to finding happiness is through acceptance of what is and can't be changed.

Rather than try to convince you of this (which might be hard if you are facing some of the issues mentioned above), maybe the best thing to do is to encourage you to just observe what happens the next time you find yourself unhappy. Chances are there will be something about the situation that you are not accepting. Ask yourself, when this happens, is there just ONE thing about the situation that I could accept—and thus make it easier to cope? When you figure out what that one thing might be—try and accept it, and see how it makes you feel.

Reinhold Niebuhr's serenity prayer has inspired many people to new heights of acceptance: *"God grant me the serenity to accept the things I cannot change, courage to change the things I can change, and wisdom to know the difference."*

When you wind up in a challenging situation, always ask yourself: *Can this situation be easily changed, or is it already done and can't be changed?* Many people feel tremendous pain about things that are already done and can't be changed. These folks are, on some level, the best candidates for applying the cure of acceptance—although they don't always see it that way. For example, when you get a speeding ticket, or are involved in a fender bender, or you lose something precious—the sooner you accept your new reality, the quicker you will recover from your pain.

Then there are times where the change is ongoing. In those situations we have to ask ourselves: *is the change worth resisting or can I just accept it?* There's a saying that applies here: *"What we resist persists."* For example, if your teenager is starting to act up and rebel a bit, that's a completely natural part of growing up. Psychologists call this individuation. You can either resist this stage in your child's development, or take it with a large dollop of acceptance. It's your choice. Resistance often exacerbates the distance between you. But acceptance often bridges the gap and eventually leads to reconciliation.

You'll almost always know when acceptance is the right path because the very minute you accept what is and can't be changed— you will feel a sense of serenity and calmness in your gut. You'll know you made the right decision. And as a result of this sensation—that you can feel in your belly and in your heart*—you will have learned how to access 'the wisdom to know the difference.'

There are millions of neurons throughout your body and many of them centered around your heart and in your gut. These neurons make heart-felt reactions and gut reactions all the more real!

"Chances are there will be something about the situation that you are not accepting. Ask yourself, when this happens, is there just ONE thing about the situation that I could accept—and thus make it easier to cope?"

❺ Keep Your Stress In Perspective

In order to keep your stress in perspective, try ranking your problems on a scale of 1-100. 1 is a broken shoelace and 100 is a nuclear holocaust. On that scale, most of our everyday stressors don't rank very high. Another method for keeping things in perspective is imagining that your hand represents a particular problem with which you are grappling. You can actually try this right now:

Flatten out your hand and hold it at arm's length. Picture that your hand is your problem and you can see it in perspective. Now slowly bring your hand right up to your nose. When you do this, about all you can see is your hand, which of course, represents your problem. (We spend much of our lives with our noses totally buried in our problems. See chapters 7 and 8.) But when you extend your arm back out, all of a sudden your problem doesn't seem so big any more. Even though the size of your problem doesn't change, you now see it in perspective—at arm's length—and it doesn't seem overwhelming anymore.

When dealing with stress, it always helps to ask yourself: how likely am I to remember this stressful situation a week from now, or a few days from now, or even a few hours from now? If the answer is not likely, then you know it's a minor problem and you could cognitively decide to let the problem go—right this minute.

Humor also really helps keep things in perspective. Humorist and stress expert, Loretta LaRoche explains *"Stress is funny!"* She likes to poke fun at herself whenever she feels stressed. "How serious is this?" She always asks herself in a delightfully lighthearted manner: "A wet towel left on the bed is NOT the same as a mugging!"

When we can laugh about our stress it takes the sting out of it. Humor author, Leigh Anne Jasheway writes about something she calls the *misery index*. She defines this as the amount time it takes to turn a stressful event or encounter with someone into a funny anecdote. If you can have something stressful happen to you in the morning on the way to work and be laughing about it by lunch time, that's a pretty short misery index. You can actually monitor and track the average amount of time it takes for you to turn an event like this around. Whether it is four days or four hours, see if you can try to find a way to laugh about a stressful incident and cut your misery index in half. It's a great goal to shoot for and will automatically help you begin to keep your stress in perspective.

When stressful problems come up at the end of the day, here's another way to keep your stress in perspective:

Promise yourself that you will tackle the problem first thing the next morning. But, here's the most important part—don't think about that problem one bit while you are away from it. Your perspective comes from TRUSTING that you will readily solve the problem the NEXT day. Overnight, your unconscious mind goes to work on solving it—especially when you're not consciously thinking about it.

You'll be surprised at all the solutions you come up with when you tackle the problem the next morning when you're fresh—simply because the next morning, you can see your problem *in the proper perspective*.

It's amazing how many different ways there are to keep your stress in perspective and yet how few people actually attempt do this. We tend to do exactly the opposite, thus creating mountains out of molehills and tempests in teapots. As shown in all the techniques in this chapter, keeping your stress in perspective is literally just a thought away. The key ingredient is building the habits that allow you to employ these techniques over and over again, whenever you have the opportunity.

The five cognitive techniques discussed in this chapter will work well for you—they only require your full commitment. You have to commit to *invoking* them at every opportunity, because every time you replace an old dysfunctional thought or behavior with a new rational thought or behavior, you create new pathways in the brain. Eventually these new pathways will become habits.

Think of this process like forging a new walking path through a field of tall grass (without the benefit of a lawnmower or a machete.) Of course it will take numerous trips before your new path will become clear, let alone permanent. But every time you invoke one of the five cognitive stress-management techniques from this chapter, you will literally be forging a new pathway in your own brain. Do it often enough and you will, without fail, forge new healthy habits that will replace your old counter-productive habits. In so doing, you'll build a whole new path to a *whole new life*. ☉

> "If you can have something stressful happen to you in the morning on the way to work and be laughing about it by lunch time, that's a pretty short misery index."

CHAPTER 5
Addicted To
Stress

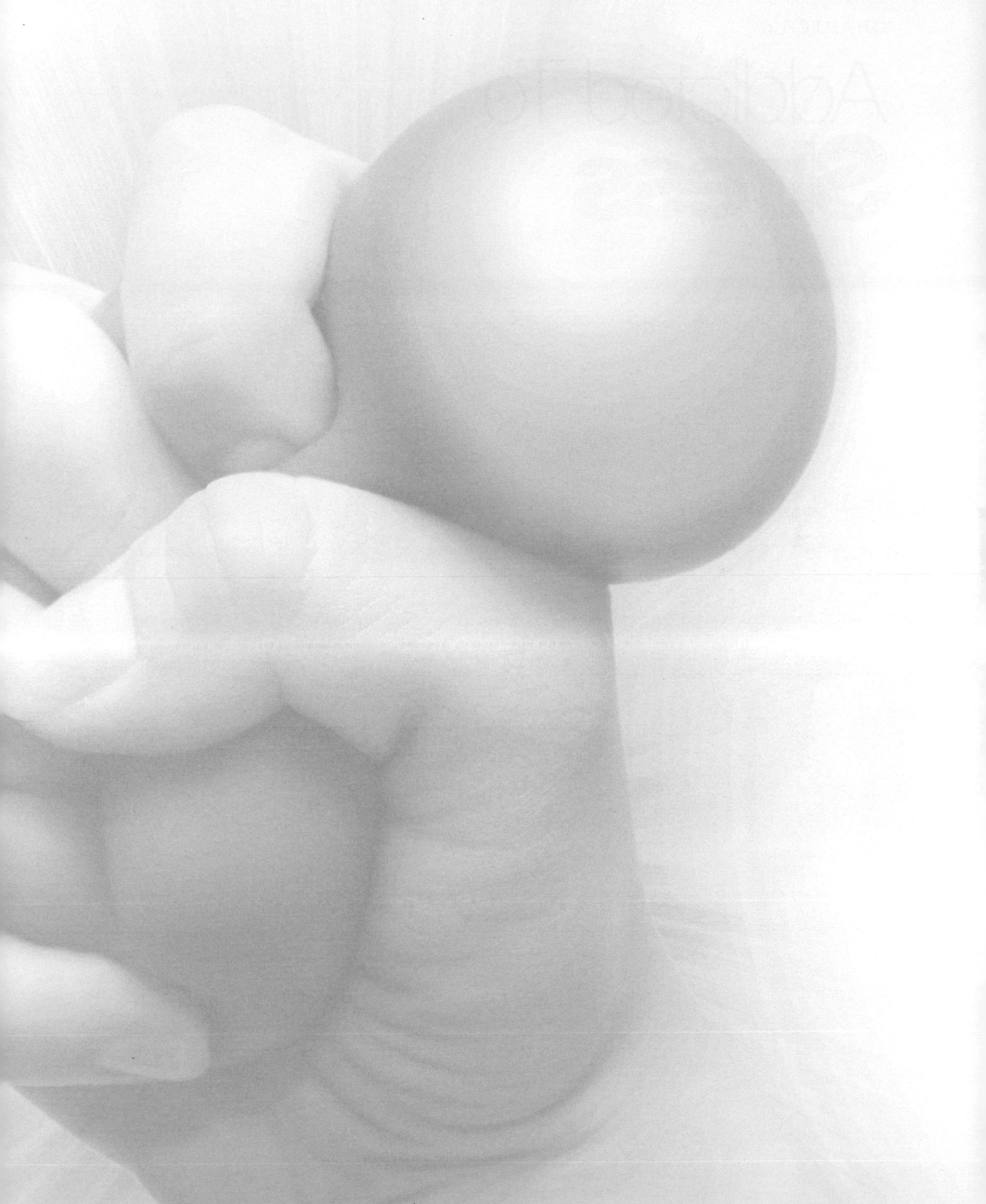

CHAPTER 5

Addicted To
Stress

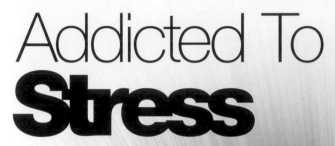

We are all somewhat addicted to stress. It's why we love excitement, roller coasters, murder mysteries and Edgar Allan Poe. We often like to feel a little scared, a little wired and a little pumped. *It tingles. It's invigorating. It's distracting.*

Stress Is A Buzz!

Every time you go to an exciting football game, dive off a high dive, see a scary movie, watch the 11 o'clock news or play a video game, your body releases small amounts of the stress chemicals adrenaline and cortisol into your blood stream. The effect these stress chemicals have on you is roughly the same as drinking a strong cup of coffee or a highly caffeinated energy drink.

Another reason why we like stress is that it actually makes us more efficient. As you can see by the graph in *Figure 1*, there's a relationship between increasing levels of stress and optimal performance—but only to a certain point.

As our level of stress or arousal increases, so does our level of performance. In other words, there's nothing like an important deadline (such as planning a wedding or getting ready for a big vacation) to get us moving and performing at our peak. But, give us too many deadlines, or a task we feel we're ill-equipped to handle, and we wind up going over the top of the curve into the red area of too much stress.

Dr. Hans Selye, who popularized the term 'stress,' once said that "stress can be the spice of life or the kiss of death." Selye had a name for the kind of stress that gets us motivated—he called this *eustress*. A hole-in-one, a promotion, getting married or having a baby are all examples of eustress.

FROM BOREDOM TO PEAK PERFORMANCE

Here's an example of how to move a mundane task up the graph—from boredom to peak performance. The next time you empty the dishwasher when it's fully loaded (a boring left-side-of-the-graph task), try this:

⏱ **Set the timer on the stove for three minutes.**

⏱ **See if you can empty the whole dishwasher before the buzzer sounds.**

⏱ **Notice how a little stress (the challenge of working against the clock) increases your productivity, focus and even enjoyment in performing an otherwise boring task.**

FIGURE 1

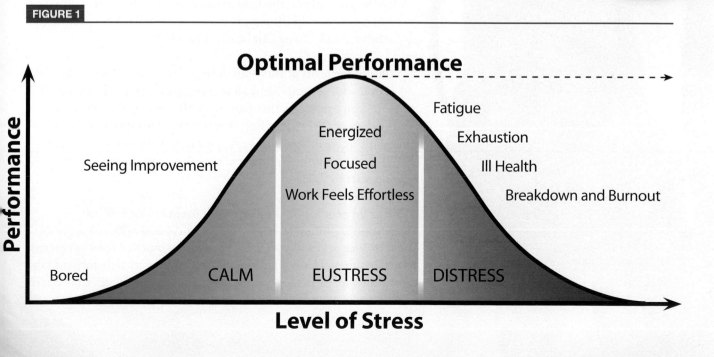

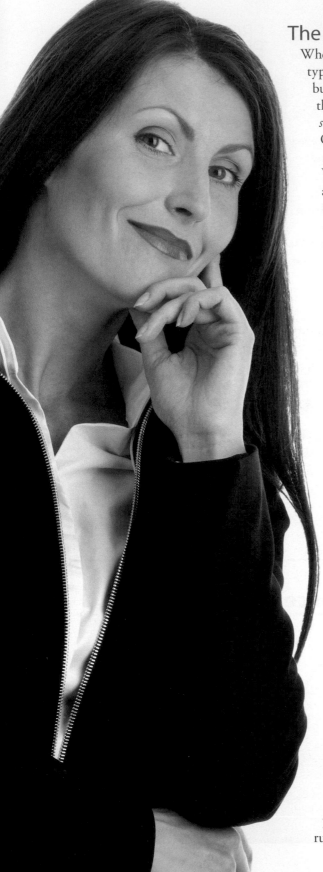

The Importance Of Eustress

When you're *glad* you're busy, you're probably experiencing eustress. This type of positive stress happens when you're operating on all cylinders, but not in any danger of breaking down. Dr. Robert Eliot, author of the book *From Stress to Strength*, called this kind of stress *N.I.C.E. stress*. NICE is an acronym for anything that is New, Interesting, Challenging or Exciting.

When we successfully multi-task, work against a deadline, feel appropriately challenged by our job or even travel somewhere for the first time, we feel this pleasant low-level sensation of stress chemicals coursing through our bloodstream. As a result, we usually feel more alive, more awake and more challenged. It spurs us on to move up the graph a little more. As long as we manage to keep all our balls in the air, we feel the rush of accomplishment and the glow of self-satisfaction.

When we feel like we are at "the top of our game," we're literally at the top of the graph, too. Perhaps you've experienced a time in your life when you couldn't believe how productive you were. Maybe there was a big project that you were really excited about. It might have been something you did in your spare time, or it might have been something you did at work. Whatever it was, it challenged you in ways you had never been challenged before. Maybe you directed a play, organized a big fundraiser, planned a large gathering, or were put in charge of an important project at work.

Sometimes, looking back, you can't believe you accomplished what you did. You endured all the stress involved in making the big decisions, getting things done and overseeing the work of friends and/or co-workers who helped you complete the project. This feeling of accomplishment is exactly what Selye was referring to when he said: "stress can be the spice of life."

One of the goals of this book is to put you back in touch with the person who accomplished all of those great things: THE TRUE YOU! You can access that person anytime you want, and as you move through the succeeding chapters you'll want to refer back to this graph as we discuss the ways you can stay on top of the curve. You'll also learn how to climb back up the graph, in the event you should start to slide.

So why do people start to slide or fall over the edge? When you were young, you probably rose up the curve and achieved optimal performance or eustress without experiencing much in the way of stress-related health problems. That's because most stress-related problems take years to develop. In fact, on your way up, you may have even enjoyed the rush of adrenaline you felt every time you experienced stress.

Losing Your Balance

However, once you're on top of the curve, this is where you can start to lose your balance because you might already believe you can take whatever stress that life throws at you. Or, you might think it's better to soldier on and ignore your stress symptoms like agitation, anger, anxiety, stomach upsets, back pain, neck pain, heart palpitations, recurrent colds and high blood pressure. Instead of taking time out to de-stress, you just keep on pushing. As your life becomes more complicated and more burdened, you may even wonder why you are unable to keep on taking it, like you could when you were younger.

This is usually the point when you start *using stress to distract yourself from stress.* This happens when you engage in mild versions of the counter-productive coping strategies that were covered in the first chapter, such as overspending, overeating and other self-sabotaging behaviors. Maybe you become "addicted" to watching CNN or Fox news, or checking your emails, or talking on your cell phone, or playing video or computer games, or driving over the speed limit. These could all be warning signs that you are heading toward ill-health, chronic fatigue, breakdown and/or burnout. In other words, the north side of that upside down U.

> "Once you're on top of the curve, this is where you can start to lose your balance because you might start thinking you can take whatever stress life throws at you."

> "When we get accustomed to a certain level of stimulation, sometimes it takes even more stimulation to distract us from our underlying sense of anxiety or agitation."

Counter-Productive Coping Skills

When we start to manage our stress in this way (by engaging in distracting but slightly stress-inducing behaviors), we get a false sense of security thinking that we are in control of them—we think that we have our hand on the spigot and can turn up or turn down the stress anytime we want. However, when we get accustomed to a certain level of stimulation, sometimes it takes even more stimulation to distract us from our underlying sense of anxiety or agitation. We don't even realize that we're distracted, so we keep compounding stress on top of the stress we're already used to—and that's when a stress number of 2 or 3 starts feeling like 0 because we are just a little stressed ALL THE TIME. In other words, we get completely accustomed to feeling a little anxious on a daily basis.

It is at this point that we can end up over-eating, over-spending, drinking too much, smoking or taking narcotics to manage our stress. We keep raising the stakes on our distracting activities just so we can keep our minds off of our ever-increasing array of problems. Craving eustress, we keep bringing more stress into our lives. As a result, we wind up causing ourselves more problems and ultimately more stress—like the gambler who eventually bankrupts himself, hoping desperately for one last big payout.

Then, we find we're caught in a vicious cycle that takes us all the way to the edge of bankruptcy, breakdown and burnout—whether that means opting for a highly risky business venture, taking on a jumbo mortgage that we can't afford, or adding something even more unsavory to our lives like developing a gambling habit or feeling like we're above the law when it comes to speed limits, traffic lights or paying taxes.

BEWARE: Addictive Behaviors That Undermine Your Health

When we talk about dealing with stress, often times we're really talking about dealing with a variety of behaviors that may not seem addictive, but actually are. Of course, there are varying degrees of addiction. Habitually using certain substances like caffeine, alcohol or tobacco to manage stress is a physical or chemical addiction—and these are the hardest addictions to overcome.

We can also become *psychologically* addicted to certain relatively harmless activities like watching TV, surfing the internet, playing video games, buying new clothes and constantly checking our hand-held electronic devices. Only YOU can tell whether these mildly addictive coping strategies may have actually risen to the level of being counter-productive by acknowledging how much time you spend doing them, and whether they actually interfere with your responsibilities at work, to your family and to yourself.

We all recognize the need to be responsible at work and toward our family, but very few of us recognize the need to be responsible to ourselves. *For most people, this is a totally foreign concept.* This simply means you must maintain your own good health— including your mental health. Let's face it, if you don't take *really good* care of yourself, you can't be a *really good* worker, a *really good* parent, or a *really good* friend.

Sometimes these slightly addicting stressful activities undermine your health in subtle ways that you're unaware of. That's because—at first—you're climbing up the curve of stress to high-performance. Eventually, though, you'll pay the consequences if you continue to treat yourself in this "irresponsible" way. You'll start to slide over the edge into breakdown and burnout, and your health *will* be negatively impacted.

Typically, we fool ourselves into thinking that this won't happen to us. That somehow we're immune to the eventual costs that MOST people pay for ignoring their stress. With that in mind, maybe it will help to examine the lifestyle of someone else—in this case, a fictional person. Let's look at a very stressful day in the life of SALLY—an average, but overly busy person who is about to slip off the top of the stress curve— and try to see if there are any similarities between her life and yours.

 www.welcoa.org

A Day In The Life Of...

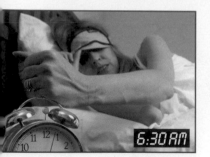

6:30 AM Sally's alarm rings. She gets up, and makes herself her first cup of coffee of the day. (*Is this a counter-productive coping strategy [CPCS]?* Only Sally can tell—based on how many MORE cups she has later—whether she is truly dependent on coffee to *wake her up*, or whether the caffeine she is consuming is causing her to stay awake at night.)

While Sally waits for the coffee to brew, she scans the paper while watching the morning news. The news is bad. To calm herself, she eats a high-carb breakfast like a bagel or an egg sandwich. (*Her second CPCS?* Sally, again, has to be the judge: Does the sandwich make her feel tired later; is she gaining a lot of weight around the middle as the result of calming herself with too many high-carb meals?)

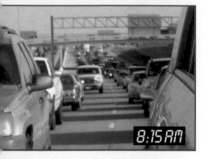

8:15 AM She gets in the car, not having left quite enough time to get to work. She feels her anxiety levels climb (her stress number) as the traffic gets more congested. When she arrives at work ten minutes late, she manages her stress by smoking a cigarette and/or sipping another cup of coffee. (*Her third and possibly fourth CPCS?*)

9:43 AM The boss appears at Sally's work station and complains about something she thought she'd done *perfectly* the day before. Sally fantasizes about quitting or doing something much worse. In order to soothe herself, she does some passive-aggressive activity like surfing the internet, checking Facebook, or making a personal call to complain about her boss to her spouse or best friend. (*Her fifth CPCS?*)

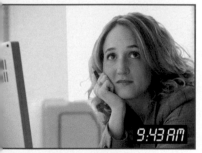

11:52 AM She uses her lunch hour to go to the doctor or the pharmacy to find something that will help with the ever-increasing back pain, neck pain, stomach pain, headache pain, depression, allergies or the recurrent colds she's been suffering from lately, and gets a prescription or over-the-counter remedy to alleviate it. Even though this coping strategy simply MASKS her stress symptoms, at least it's doctor approved! (*Her sixth CPCS?*)

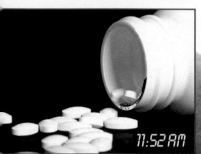

12:57 PM On her way back to the office, Sally stops at a fast food restaurant and over-rides her better judgment by ordering a burger, fries and a shake. Even though that large vanilla shake has over 1,000 calories, she savors every last drop because it seems to soothe her emotionally. (*Her seventh CPCS?*)

(Continued on next page) ▶

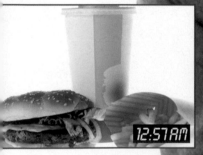

Stressed-Out Sally

1:23 PM   Back at work, *another* boss comes by and gives her an assignment that conflicts with her first assignment. She's not sure which one is more important, so she takes a cigarette break while she decides what to do, or just reads a business publication that looks like it's work related. *(Her eighth CPCS?)* She decides to work on what the second boss wants until her first boss walks in at 5:00 PM and wonders why she hasn't finished the first assignment. She works overtime until both assignments are done.

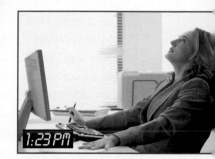

6:42 PM   She was planning on going for a walk after work, but it's already dark, so Sally just grabs a glass of wine, a block of cheese and opens a box of low fat crackers, which she calls dinner. *(Her ninth and tenth CPCS?)* She sits down in front of the TV and watches a reality show that she's mildly addicted to. *(Her eleventh CPCS?)*

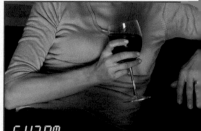

7:15 PM   She feels like another glass of wine or at least some ice cream, but she decides to go to the mall instead. She notices her mood shift a bit as she walks around the mall and moves her body. She actually starts feeling a little better and resists the urge to eat a cookie the size of her head, and opts to browse in a clothing store instead. She finds the perfect outfit for work and decides to buy it even though it's a bit pricey. When the cashier hands her back her credit card and says her purchase has been declined—in front of five other people waiting—Sally heads right back to that cookie place and eats that oversized cookie in three bites. *(Her twelfth CPCS?)*

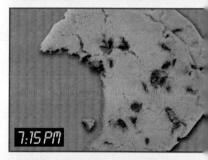

10:15 PM   When she finally gets back home and lays in bed, she's so wired that she decides to stay up and watch the 11 o'clock news.

12:00 AM   When she turns the TV off around midnight, she realizes she's still not tired at all, so she takes a sleeping pill. *(Her unlucky thirteenth CPCS of the day?* As before, Sally has to be the judge of what she's doing. Most doctors prescribe sleeping pills to get you through a stressful period. They don't want you to become dependent on them. So if Sally IS dependent on them, and she's been taking them for months or even years, then yes, this is a CPCS.)

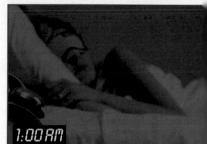

1:00 AM   She finally falls asleep.

6:30 AM   Sally's alarm goes off to start another day.

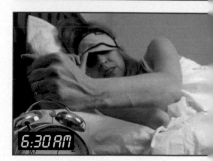

HOW DOES YOUR TYPICAL DAY COMPARE TO SALLY'S?

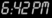   If you've ever had a day or parts of your day that are this stressful, you are going to spend those waking hours and minutes with your internal organs bathing in stress hormones. If it only happens once in a while, it's no big deal. Your body can fully recover from occasional episodes of stress. But if your stress is chronic, over time, this unrelenting hormonal assault can do damage to your blood vessels, your kidneys, your digestive tract, your heart, your memory and it will speed up the aging process, too. Spend enough days, months and years living like this and eventually it's likely to raise your blood pressure, increase your (resting) heart rate, cause you to overeat—and can eventually lead to all kinds of MAJOR health problems like diabetes, heart disease and stroke.

ADDICTED TO TV:

So how do we know when our love of something, whether it's texting, playing video games or just watching TV, has turned into a mild form of addiction? The California State University at Northridge reports the following information about TV addiction on their website:

"Millions of Americans are so hooked on television that they fit the criteria for substance abuse as defined in the official psychiatric manual. Heavy TV viewers exhibit five dependency symptoms—two more than necessary to arrive at a clinical diagnosis of substance abuse. These include:

1. **Using TV as a sedative.**

2. **Indiscriminate viewing.**

3. **Feeling loss of control while viewing.**

4. **Feeling angry with oneself for watching too much.**

5. **Inability to stop watching.**

6. **Feeling miserable when kept from watching."**

Usually, addictive behaviors disrupt peoples' lives, are difficult to stop and people use them as an escape from their troubles. It is these very real consequences that turn an ordinary behavior into a mild form of addiction or at the very least, a counter-productive coping strategy.

Maintaining Your Balance

Nobody wants to put themselves at risk for all these health problems, but very few people understand the importance of maintaining BALANCE at the top of the stress curve. Usually, by the time we realize something is wrong—that we are sliding down the far side of curve—we are often so addicted to our stressful coping behaviors that it FEELS like it's impossible to change them.

Changing behaviors, especially deeply engrained counter-productive coping strategies you've relied on for years like drinking, smoking, drug-taking, overeating and overspending, can be a more difficult process than just changing your thoughts. But as we've said before, ANY behavioral change is possible. You just need to know HOW to change. The good news is: there's one psychologist from Rhode Island who's figured out something about change that no one else has.

Want to know what it is? Read the next chapter to find out.

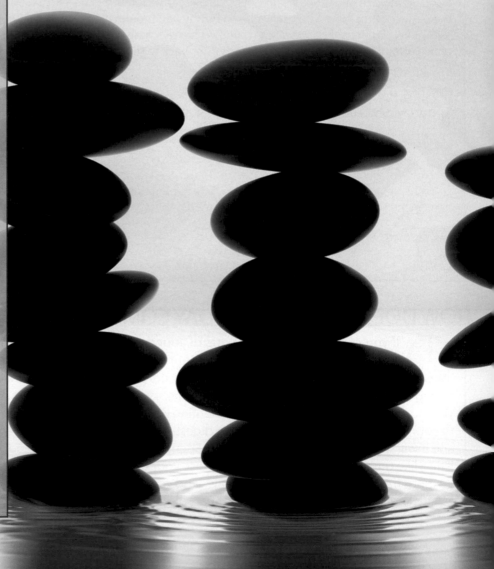

www.welcoa.org

"Stress can be the spice of life or the kiss of death."

—Dr. Hans Selye

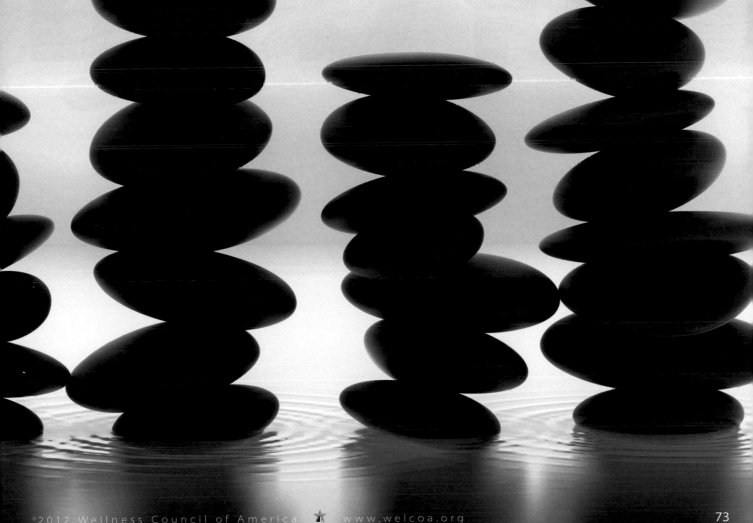

CHAPTER 6

Changing Your Behavior
For Good

nge For Good

O ACTION PLAN NOW

CHAPTER 6

Changing Your Behavior
For Good

Thirty years ago, Dr. James Prochaska, a psychologist at the University of Rhode Island, began studying how people change. What he learned about behavioral change has helped thousands and thousands of people quit smoking and end other unhealthy behaviors who might not have done so without his brilliant research.

Prochaska discovered that change takes place in stages. People need to work up to changing and learn about changing before launching any new behavior. That may sound obvious, but if you try to throw yourself right into a change program, or what Prochaska calls the "action stage" (like an exercise plan, a smoking cessation class or a diet) before you're fully ready, you will inevitably fail.

This was a key finding since most programs typically START in the action phase. Prochaska determined that everyone, whether they realize it or not, goes through five stages before they can turn an unhealthy habit into a healthy one.

> When you decide what it is you want to change, or the new habit you want to add in, start small. Make one change at time and practice it for weeks, if not months, before adding in additional layers of change.

The Five Stages Of Behavior Change

1. In the first stage, you simply become aware of the need to change. *(Back in the 1950s, few people had any idea that smoking was harmful, so in the 1960s the government started insisting that tobacco companies put health warnings on cigarettes.)*

2. In the second stage, you learn about *why* you should change. *(The government soon realized that just telling people that smoking "was hazardous to your health" wasn't enough to get them to quit. That's in part why government agencies heavily funded Prochaska's research, which began in the 1970s.)* What Prochaska discovered was that people need LOTS of reasons why they should quit, such as: you will live longer, your house won't smell of smoke, your breath won't smell of smoke, your teeth will be whiter, you'll be able to climb stairs without panting, you'll be less agitated, you'll sleep better, you'll save thousands of dollars and, of course, your spouse, your children and even your dog WON'T develop lung cancer from exposure to second hand smoke.

3. In the third stage, you consider *how* you want to change. This is where you develop a plan of action for exactly what you are going to do next. For smokers, developing a plan of action usually involves talking to your doctor, talking to friends who have successfully quit, finding support groups and/or programs, or getting a prescription for a patch—all of which will help you feel *confident* about your ability to change. Only after you've moved through these first three stages—where you've become AWARE of the problem, learned all about WHY you should change and developed a PLAN of action—are you actually ready to *take* ACTION (Stage 4.)

4. In the fourth stage, you take action: carrying out the plan—that up to now— you've been only thinking about. (For smokers, it might be you simply smoke one or two less cigarettes per day, keeping careful track of the exact number. Your plan would eventually take you down to zero cigarettes a day over the course of weeks or months.)

5. The fifth stage is where you try to MAINTAIN your healthy behaviors. This is the crucial step where you usually need some help to keep from falling off the wagon. People seldom realize that *RELAPSE IS PART OF THE PROCESS*. Prochaska's research shows that smokers typically relapse three or four times before finally quitting for good. It's important to realize this so you don't beat yourself up unmercifully when you inevitably take a step backwards.

Prochaska often points out: the biggest reason why people relapse is STRESS. Some stressful event like getting into an accident, a nasty argument, or breaking up with one's significant other will upset the apple cart and the person defaults to their old counter-productive coping strategy (in order to cope with the stress.) So, according to Prochaska, people aren't likely to achieve any form of behavioral change without some kind of rock-solid stress management program already in place. (Look no further than the confines of this book!)

Life Events Are Launching Pads

One of the surprisingly simple motivators for change is a life event. People often quit smoking or start eating healthier when they have a baby, or move in with or marry someone who *doesn't* smoke or who eats vegetarian—or even when they have an accidental interruption in their old habit, say, in the case of an illness such as bronchitis where they don't feel like smoking for a certain period of time. All these life events can help you end a bad habit and launch a new one.

To share a personal example: My father had his tonsils out as an adult, just after the surgeon general's warning started appearing on cigarettes. He didn't feel like smoking for about three weeks, and he knew from educating himself (Stage 2) that he was over the hard part. My mother gave up smoking too, in order to give him moral support. This is exactly the way life events can be a springboard for behavioral change.

My parents were further motivated by not wanting me or my older brothers to smoke. This is another great motivator for making any therapeutic lifestyle change: *doing it for someone else.* Getting people to think about what they truly value in life (like family, or generosity, or love) gets them in touch with making lifestyle changes that support those values. Many people value family more than anything. And imagining what they are leaving their children or grandchildren in terms of a legacy (like smoking versus a healthier lifestyle) can really motivate one to make a positive lifestyle change.

WHAT WE OFTEN VALUE

- ⏰ Family
- ⏰ Success
- ⏰ Happiness
- ⏰ Integrity
- ⏰ Freedom
- ⏰ Religion
- ⏰ God
- ⏰ Money
- ⏰ Health
- ⏰ Fame

Spending some time thinking about what you really value in life is an important exercise. Once you do this, you may discover that how you spend the bulk of your time is not in harmony with your highest values. For example, if your highest value is family and you work 60+ hours a week, you're going to feel a lot of inner conflict, even if you are simply working to pay for all the things your family wants and needs.

My Top Five Values Are:

❶
❷
❸
❹
❺

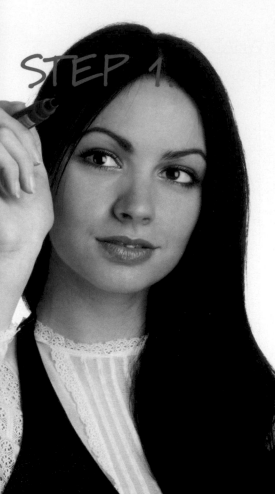

STEP 1

Focus On What's Important To You

Do you want your children (or your nieces and nephews) to be smokers? Do you want your children to be overweight? Do you want your children to be as stressed as you are? Of course, you don't. But when you model this behavior, you are greatly increasing the odds of passing it along to the next generation. And even if you are single, do you want people to remember you (or think of you) as a stressed out, angry person? Chances are, you don't.

When considering changing your habits around stress, ask yourself: *what if my own "peace of mind" was really my highest value? Would I keep the same job? Would I work as much overtime? Would I have as high a mortgage? Would I spend more time with my family?* Really studying your values can help you motivate yourself to make BIG lifestyle changes. (See chart on the previous page.)

Another way to facilitate change is by asking yourself, on a scale of 1–10, *how important is it for me to make this change?* The next question you should ask yourself is: *on a scale of 1–10, how confident am I in my ability to make a change?*

Your answers to these two questions may give you an idea of where you are in the stages of change and whether you're ready for the action stage. You need to have a high degree of confidence and give the change you want to make a high level of importance if you hope to be successful. If you find yourself answering either question with a LOW number, ask yourself the additional question: *what would it take to get my confidence a few points higher on the readiness scale?*

> "When considering changing your habits around stress, ask yourself: what if my own "peace of mind" was really my highest value?"

Get Ready To Take Action

Prochaska discovered that in any given population of people wishing to change, ONLY about 20% are ready to take *action* and 80% want to change but ARE NOT ready to take action—yet. Take a careful look at yourself. Are YOU in that 80% who is only *thinking* about change? If so, learn before you leap. Find out *more* about lowering stress, about quitting smoking or about taking up exercise. Hold back on taking action until your knowledge of the pros of launching this new behavior *thoroughly outweigh* the cons of giving it up.

In other words, if you are currently in Stage 1, you will need to learn a lot more about why you should change and how you should change before jumping into the action stage, or you will most likely FAIL and blame yourself for your lack of willpower. Remember: as Prochaska's research shows, it's NOT NECESSARILY LACK OF WILLPOWER, but rather, *inadequate readiness to change that causes us to fail.*

Five Simple Steps To Less Stress

Perhaps the reason that Prochaska's stages of change are not more widely known is that, generally, he appeals to health professionals and speaks in their language. Therefore, I've taken the liberty of simplifying some of his terminology to make the stages of change easier for you to understand.

All behavioral change begins with awareness of what it is you want to change. So *awareness* of the problem is Step 1. Step 2 is to learn *why you want to make a change.* Step 3 is to decide *how you want to change,* i.e., to come up with a plan. Step 4 is to put your plan into *action.* And Step 5 is to *maintain* your plan despite any setbacks you may encounter. And that's it.

Step 1. **Awareness** of what it is you want to change.

Step 2. Learning **why** you want to make a change.

Step 3. Deciding **how** you want to make a change. (Come up with a plan.)

Step 4. Putting your plan into **action**.

Step 5. **Maintaining** your plan despite any relapses that may occur.

It's probably safe to assume that if you've read this far, you have some stressful behaviors you'd like to change. Maybe it's a counter-productive coping strategy like smoking, or maybe you'd like to simply begin meditating or exercising to reduce your stress. No matter what the behavior you want to adopt or change, it will help you to know how the stages of change work specifically in regards to reducing stress.

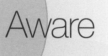

1 Aware

2 Why

3 How

4 Action

5 Transform

How To Reduce Your Stress In Stages

STAGE 1 **You become AWARE that you have stress and that it might be a good idea to lower it.** You think that, *yes it's really unhealthy for me to push myself all the time and maybe I do need to do something about lowering my stress.* You've been getting headaches and feeling short-tempered with your kids or your friends and co-workers, and you wonder if reducing stress might help.

STAGE 2 **You determine WHY you want to lower your stress.** Here you find out that YES, stress is associated with headaches, agitation and anger. So you start weighing the pros and cons of actually making a change: *If I took up exercise, meditation or yoga, that would take time—but it would be well worth it if I could get over my migraine headaches and not alienate my friends with my moodiness.* You find out a lot of other good reasons to lower stress, including: reducing your risk of certain kinds of chronic pain, allergies, gastrointestinal problems, high blood pressure, heart disease, diabetes and stroke.

STAGE 3 **You figure out HOW you are going to lower your stress.** You select the method or program you are going to participate in. You come up with a plan. You talk to friends or experts (like your doctor) who give you some advice about what options are available to you. Perhaps your best friend convinces you to sign up for a yoga or a meditation class, or maybe you find a gym, a personal exercise trainer, or even a walking buddy to help you start putting your plan into place.

STAGE 4 **You take ACTION and begin to exercise, meditate or do yoga.** In the action stage, it's always a good idea to start small. Pick a target that you know you can easily reach. That way, you will experience some initial success, right off the bat. Even doing something as little as 15 minutes a day can help you successfully launch a new habit like exercising, meditating or doing yoga.

STAGE 5 **You TRANSFORM your goal into a habit, understanding that you'll experience a few set-backs along the way.** Change doesn't occur in a continuous forward motion. You often have a few set-backs. So, the key to making it over the finish line and into the final stage is learning how to forgive yourself for any relapses that occur.

In the final stage, you come to the unshakable conclusion that it is better to maintain your new habit than to give it up. In other words, now that you rarely get migraine headaches anymore and you are much less moody and can communicate better with your friends, there's no way you are going to go back to your old ways and give up your now regular practice of yoga, meditation or exercise.

Abstinence Violation Effect

There's one more thing you'll want to note: psychologists have identified a phenomenon called abstinence violation effect or AVE for short. Even after weeks or months of successfully maintaining a change, you may have a single setback that you feel so guilty about, you'll want to throw in the towel and give up all your hard work. This is AVE. Be on the lookout for this. Recognize it when it comes and gently guide yourself back into your new behavior as if you'd never left it, so you can keep moving on toward your desired result.

> "Recognize AVE (abstinence violation effect) when it comes and gently guide yourself back into your new behavior as if you'd never left it, so you can keep moving on toward your desired result."

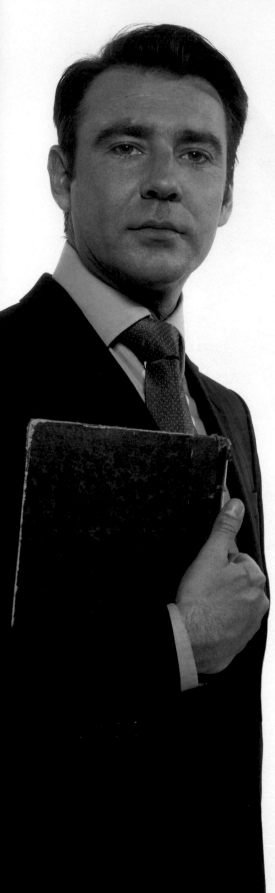

Try These On For Size

In closing out this chapter on behavioral change, here are five simple behavioral changes that you can initiate fairly easily to bring about an immediate lowering of stress in your life. With simple ideas like these—that don't require a big commitment—you can learn how to reduce your stress by simply trying these exercises for one day. You'll see results immediately and you can build your change based on the positive feedback you will experience from starting small.

1. **Stop rushing.** We rush around everywhere we go. We're almost addicted to it. Try spending one day where you don't rush anywhere. Get up earlier than you need to. Allow extra time for doing everything. Enjoy JUST ONE DAY at a leisurely pace—even if it's your day off—and see how absolutely delicious it feels to stop and chat whenever you feel like it, or to drive sanely between destinations, or to pause when the feeling moves you and literally *stop and smell the roses*.

2. **Arrive early.** In attempting to arrive places on-time, we're often late because we don't build in extra time for traffic jams, accidents and other inevitable delays. When you plan to arrive *early*, you not only allow for these unforeseen circumstances, but your travel time becomes infinitely more enjoyable because you're not spending the entire trip stressing about being late.

3. **Create a comfortable morning routine.** When you start off your day arguing with your spouse or roommate, hurrying your children or family members and trying to get yourself dressed and ready in a short period of time, you will almost certainly begin your day feeling stressed. To prevent this from happening, get things ready the night before: put out your clothes for the next day, make your lunch, take a shower before bed. Do anything you can do ahead of time, so your morning "rush" won't be so jam-packed.

4. **Go to bed earlier and <u>don't</u> watch the 11 o'clock news.** The 11 o'clock news is full of stories that are designed to catch your attention by making you feel anxious about crime, or rising prices, or storms headed your way. This is not good for your serenity and is antithetical to feeling sleepy. Turn off the TV and go to bed an hour earlier—or read something inspirational or meditate and think about everything you have to be grateful for. You'll sleep easier for it.

5. **Get organized.** Disorganization can make you "crazy." Always losing things, working from a messy desk and feeling bad about your messy house will take its toll on your sanity. Spend at least one day a month simply organizing your life. Or the next time you can't

www.welcoa.org ⭐ ©2012 Wellness Council of America

find something, instead of wasting time feeling frustrated and looking everywhere for it, just start cleaning and organizing your space. You'll probably spend about the same amount of time cleaning up as you would have wasted searching for the lost item. *And you'll almost always find the lost item in the process.*

Remember, all change begins with awareness of what it is you want to change. That's Step 1. Sit down and really analyze what is causing you the most stress. Look at your counter-productive coping strategies. Make a list of your top ten stressors. Keep a daily journal of all your stressful incidents for a few weeks and look for the names of people, activities and times of day that keep popping up. These stressful themes running through your life may be the things you want to change first.

When you decide what it is you want to change, or the new habit you want to add in, start small. Make one change at a time and practice it for weeks, if not months, before adding in additional layers of change. That way, you will ensure your eventual success. And even if you experience a setback, remember that setbacks are a part of the process. Get right back on that bucking horse named CHANGE and keep riding her until you reach the finish line where you will not be the least bit tempted to go back to your old ways. ◷

"Remember, all change begins with awareness of what it is you want to change."

CHAPTER 7

Stress Is A Word That Stands For Problems

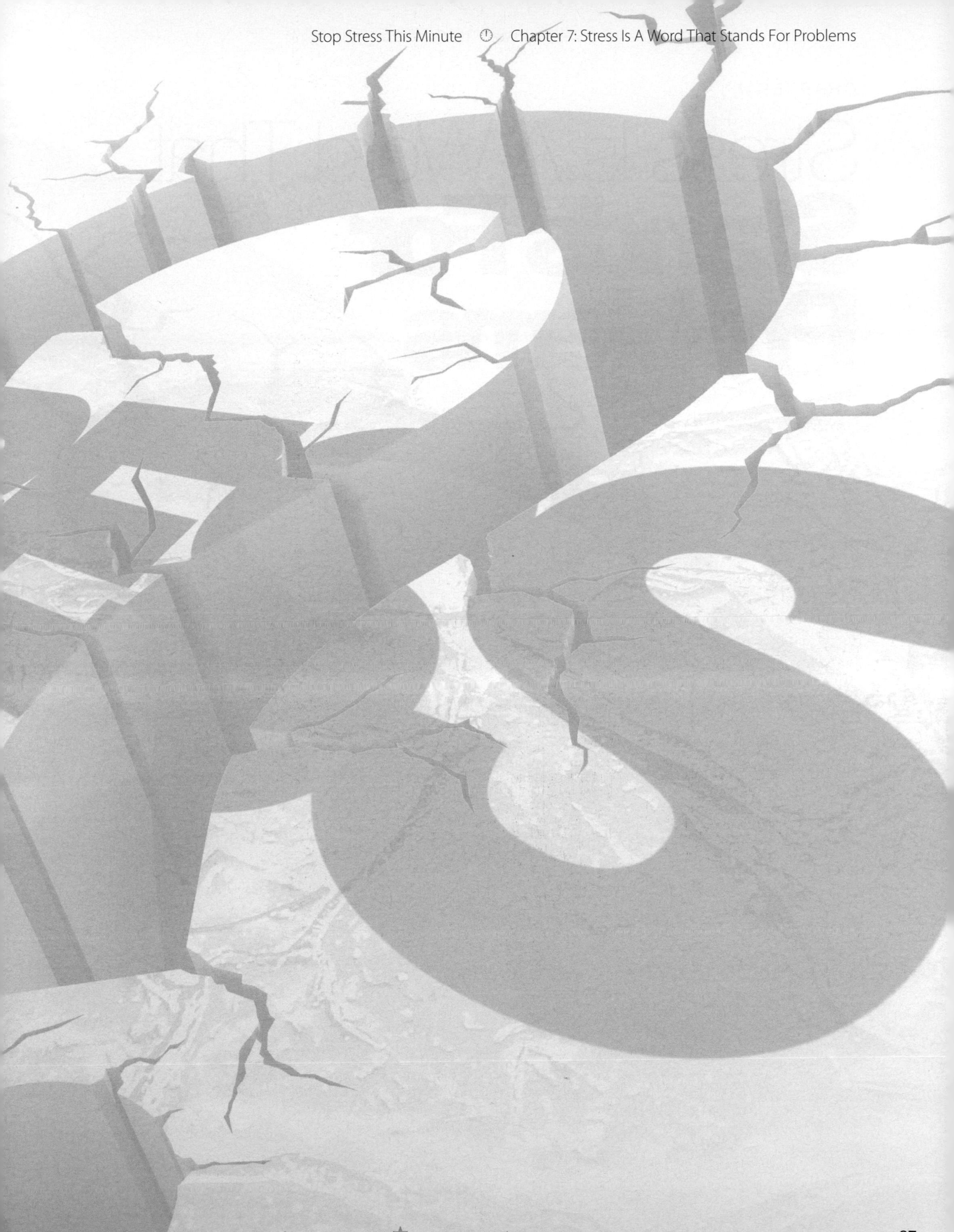

CHAPTER 7

Stress Is A Word That Stands For Problems

I n his book, *The 14-Day Stress Cure,* **Mort Orman MD makes the point that we get confused by the term stress.** Dr. Orman thinks it is kind of a vague, ubiquitous, all-inclusive term that makes stress seem like it's impossible to solve.

"You see, 'stress' is just a word we use to stand for hundreds of specific problems in our lives," Orman explained in a radio interview. "*Stress* itself is never our problem. It's just a 'buzzword' or a code word for lots of other things that trouble us. But when we lump our problems together and call them 'stress,' we forget what we really want is relief from very specific things—like getting angry, feeling frustrated, having bad relationships or dealing with all sorts of other day-to-day problems."

"So if we got rid of the word, *which of course we're not going to do*, or if we keep reminding ourselves that stress means problems, I think we would all be much better off. Then, instead of asking: *how can I learn to deal with my stress?*, we would be forced to ask ourselves more focused questions, such as *how can I deal with anger or frustration more successfully?*; *how can I deal with a marriage that's not satisfying to me*; or *how can I deal with the fear that I might lose my job or that I'm going to get fired, or that my boss doesn't like me?* These are all much more empowering types of questions, and once you start asking them, you're in much better position to identify the causes of your problems and deal with these causes successfully."

Dr. Orman makes a very good point. The word stress generalizes our problems to the point where we don't really have to face each problem individually and figure out how to solve it. In this chapter, we're going to take a problem-solving approach to learning how to manage stress. We're going to show you how to tease apart your stressful dilemmas into identifiable problems you can analyze and solve, one problem at a time. We've broken this process down into the following five steps.

❶ Identify it.

❷ Analyze it.

❸ Solve it.

❹ Put your plan into action.

❺ Stay with the plan.

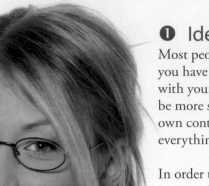

❶ Identify It

Most people think that Step 1 is a "no-brainer." But simply telling yourself you have a lot of stress (even if you narrow it down to the stress you have with your boss or your spouse or your finances) is too vague. You need to be more specific. You need to identify each stressor as it comes along in its own context. The best way to accomplish this is to keep careful track of everything that bothers you and why, for at least one week, preferably two.

In order to do this, you'll need to carry around a small, spiral notebook in your pocket, or use your day-planner or PDA to write down short notes about stressors that occur to you as they happen. For example:

8:00 AM	The kids were dawdling so I yelled at them and felt guilty.
8:30 AM	Got stuck in traffic and felt frustrated.
9:30 AM	My boss criticized my work and that made me feel angry and defensive.
7:00 AM–10:00 AM	Drank three cups of coffee today and felt anxious all afternoon.
12:30 PM	Waited in a really long line at the bank, and nearly blew my top when the teller refused to cash my check.
1:30 PM	Left my credit card at a restaurant and felt frantic.

In Step 1, you simply identify each *activating event* (any event that causes you stress), the time it occurred and how you *felt* afterwards.

Get A Perspective On Your Stress

If you have time at the end of the day, you can turn your log into a journal and write more about how you felt and how this affected your day. Journaling is very therapeutic—it helps you put your stress in perspective and will definitely help you vent your frustration and anger in a healthy, non-violent way. But if you don't have time for journaling (in other words, elaborating on what bugs you), just keep up with your simple log for two weeks, jotting down stressful episodes as soon after they occur as possible.

At the end of the two weeks you will undoubtedly see the names of people, activities and things popping up, day after day. You'll make connections that you wouldn't have made otherwise without the benefit of this *perspective.* You may realize that it's a certain time of day—like the morning

www.welcoa.org ★ ©2012 Wellness Council of America

rush—where you experience the most stress. You may see that it's a certain person—like your boss, or a coworker, or a relative that keeps popping up. Or you may notice some recurring aspect of unrelated activities, such as being in noisy, crowded places or tight spaces that *predictably* cause you to feel stressed.

When I kept a log several years ago, at the end of the first week, I noticed that I had experienced stress at the DMV, the bank and the grocery store. At first I didn't see the connection, but then I remembered that in each place, I had been waiting in a long line. I had always thought the DMV was just a stressful place but apparently, it was actually the waiting in line that was the true source of my distress.

I guarantee that if you keep a log or a journal for at least a week, preferably two, you will have similar "aha" experiences. If you don't want to keep a log, simply try to tackle one stressful problem per day by utilizing the remaining steps outlined below.

Stop Stress This Minute: Stress Journal

DATE/TIME	INCIDENT	DESCRIPTION

www.welcoa.org   ©2011 Wellness Council of America

This sample journal page can be found in the appendix on page 138. Please copy it and keep track of your stress.

> "The best way to identify each stressor is to keep careful track of everything that bothers you and why, for at least one week, preferably two."

❷ Analyze It

The next step is to decide what kind of stress it is you are dealing with. There's **second-hand stress**. That's when someone else is stressed and you catch it from them. There's **avoidable stress**, where, if you just did things a little differently, you could probably avoid this source of stress altogether. There's **underlying stress**, where the real source of your stress is something hidden below the surface of a more obvious cause. There's **anticipatory stress**, the stress you experience just thinking about an upcoming event. And finally, there's **unavoidable stress** that you sometimes just have to put up with and endure.

Look over your log and think carefully about what type of stress you are dealing with. Is it avoidable or unavoidable? Sometimes the answer isn't so obvious. For example, if you have a family to support and/or a monthly rent or mortgage payment to make, you will of course need to maintain your primary source of income, so dealing with a difficult boss or situation at work may be *unavoidable*. On the other hand, if that boss is making your life miserable, you may need to make some kind of change for the sake of your mental health. The takeaway here is that even some unavoidable problems, if serious enough, can and should be avoided.

However, many things that cause us stress can simply be avoided or even delegated to someone else that isn't bothered by the stress as much as we are. For instance, if you really hate waiting in line at the bank, give that job to someone else or do your banking online. The key point here is that until you sit down and analyze each problem in this way, you may not realize that there is a substantial amount of *unnecessary* stress you can simply avoid.

Dealing With Your Underlying Causes Of Stress

Dr. Orman also talks about *underlying* causes of stress. Sometimes when we analyze a stressful event, it seems like one specific thing is causing the problem (like a traffic jam, a jammed printer, a missed connection on a plane trip, or kids dawdling.) But when we look a little deeper, we see that the *underlying* cause of stress in all these examples is probably time pressure. Understanding the underlying source of stress helps you understand how to solve the problem, because you deal with time pressure *differently than you would with dawdling children*.

And that's true of all types of stress. Each kind of stress, whether it's *anticipatory, underlying, secondhand, avoidable* or *unavoidable* must be dealt with in different ways. We'll look at that in more detail in Step 3.

You also need to analyze the frequency and the severity of the problem. If it's a problem that's recurring five times a day, it is obviously going to have a different priority than if it's happening once a week.

STRESS ANALYSIS

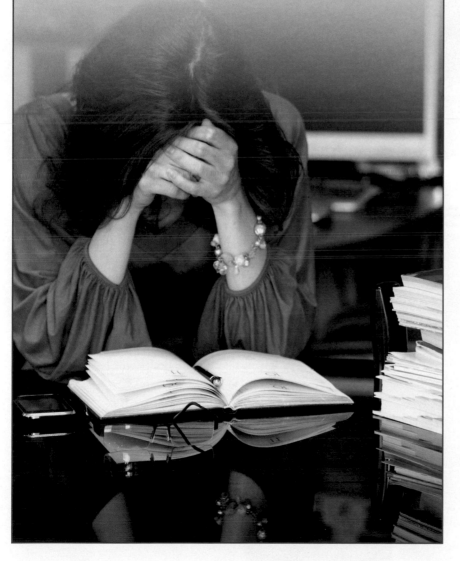

When I was first starting out in my career, I had a job I really liked, but a boss who was really difficult. I stuck around for eight years, however, because, when I *analyzed* it, I was able to see that I had about one difficult encounter with her per week. I also noted that this was usually the result of second-hand stress—in other words, it was *her stress* and not mine—and that the severity of the encounters were usually moderate to low.

Until I analyzed the type of stress plus the frequency and the severity of it, I wouldn't have realized how truly manageable my stress actually was.

"Understanding the underlying source of stress helps you understand how to solve the problem, because you deal with time pressure differently than you would with dawdling children."

"Stress is pervasive. It sneaks up on you when you're not looking, and sometimes over the silliest things."

❸ Solve It

Once you have broken down your stress into the different types, it becomes easier to solve. So let's take a closer look at each type of stress: avoidable stress, underlying stress, anticipatory stress, second hand stress and unavoidable stress.

Avoidable stress. When your stress is avoidable, or unnecessary, it's usually easy to solve. When I discovered that I was stressed by long lines at the bank, the grocery store and the DMV, I said to myself: *how can I solve this problem?* The bank was easy—just avoid Fridays at lunch hour and the end of the day. The DMV was trickier. It seemed like the lines there were always long. So, I called the DMV and found out what I needed to know— don't go at the beginning or the end of the month and don't go on Mondays or Saturdays. Midweek and mid-month are usually the best bet. *Problem identified; problem analyzed; problem solved.*

Always losing things is another source of stress that you can readily avoid. *Just get organized.* Forcing yourself to do this isn't easy, but you will eliminate a lot of unnecessary stress by simply working from an organized desk, driving in a neat and clean car, organizing your files and always putting away things like your wallet and keys in the same place every time.

Other areas of avoidable stress could include your commute (request flex hours), the morning rush (get things ready the night before), a difficult client (hand him or her over to someone else), and even a long list of household chores (*delegate* chores to your spouse and children and *don't be so picky about how they get done.*) You can't figure out what's avoidable until you identify your stress, analyze it and take the time to solve it.

Time To Get Organized!

Second-hand stress. A lot of our stress is what I call second-hand stress. It really belongs to the other person, not you. Let's say your boss or coworker comes in to work in a bad mood and then attempts to rub that mood off on you. It's often possible to see this coming, but we seldom act on our intuition and stay out of the way, or at the very least, take what is said with a grain of salt. Instead, we hear a critical tone in the other person's voice and we either get defensive or argumentative, or take the criticism to heart.

Now, if your coworker or boss is *frequently* taking things out on you, that's not good. But if it only happens once in awhile and you can give this person a *free pass* for being occasionally grumpy or rude, YOU ARE THE ONE WHO WILL BENEFIT. Just ignore the behavior—particularly if it's out of character—and you will feel a sense of *empowerment* for having done so.

Anticipatory stress. As Stanford professor and stress expert, Dr. Robert Sapolsky often says, the reason zebras don't get stress-related diseases and humans do is that zebras don't think about the lion when it's *not there*. We humans, on the other hand, can imagine lions everywhere. We think about our problems when they aren't even there. Sometimes that comes in handy—when we stock our refrigerators before a hurricane—but often times it just causes us to worry excessively and feel anxious about a lot of stuff that NEVER comes to pass.

Be aware of when your THINKING is causing you to feel stressed about events that are far off or may never even happen. *This is anticipatory stress.* And whenever this type of stress bothers you, refer back to some of the cognitive restructuring techniques that we talked about in Chapter 4.

Underlying stress. Whenever you're stuck in traffic, or something doesn't work right, or you discover you have a flat tire and you're starting to feel stressed, ask yourself: *is it the OBVIOUS problem that's making me feel stressed or is it some other underlying (or non-obvious) source of stress like time pressure?*

Time pressure is a MAJOR source of stress, yet we tend to fool ourselves into thinking it's a more obvious culprit like getting stuck in a traffic jam. As a result, we erroneously blame our stress on dawdling children, broken equipment or heavy traffic, when really it's time pressure that's putting us in a bind.

There's a simple way to deal with time pressure—build in extra time for things to go wrong or for things that take longer than you think. When you wait 'til the last day to buy all the things you need for a party, invariably, the store is going to be out of the one thing you need most. That's why you need to always build in extra time for things to go wrong (which in this case would mean not waiting until the day of the party to do your shopping.) Shop ahead of time and not only will you enjoy the shopping trip, but if there's something you don't find you'll have plenty of time to go get it somewhere else.

QUARTZ

30

Arriving at your destination well ahead of time will make your whole trip a lot less stressful. Whenever I have an important business appointment, I try to get there at least an hour or even two hours early (depending on how far away it is.) I go to the destination, find out exactly where I have to park, where the front entrance is and what floor my meeting is on. Then I go and have a leisurely breakfast or lunch, preferably within walking distance, so I know that I can make it back without any hassle or delays.

If nothing unforeseen happens, I'm able to put my extra time to good use by having a meal or reading, or checking my messages or emails in a wireless hotspot. But, if I do get stuck in some terrible traffic jam, or get hopelessly lost on the way there, I'm covered because *I've built in extra time for things to go wrong or to take longer than I had anticipated.*

Other classic areas of underlying stress include relationship problems and financial stress. When you're going through a difficult time in your relationship—or you get into an argument with your spouse on the way to work—notice how this can affect your whole day. You may find that you're more argumentative or just a little less patient, or more sensitive to criticism. Things bother you at work that normally wouldn't. Without carefully analyzing your stress, you'd probably never guess that your workday stress and your underlying relationship problems are the least bit connected.

Also, watch out for financial problems that can keep you awake in the middle of the night. The next day you'll blame your tiredness and any resultant crankiness on lack of sleep, but here again, it's not the obvious culprit, insomnia, but the *underlying* financial stress that *caused* the insomnia.

Unavoidable stress. Some stress is truly unavoidable. You just have to endure it whether that's an illness, a death in the family, getting laid-off or having trouble with your kids. Don't despair if a lot of your stress falls into this category. Learning how to handle this stress will make you more resilient in the long run. Overcoming your problems makes you into a stronger person. Face your problems head on and use everything you've learned in this book to keep this unavoidable stress within manageable limits.

> "Some stress is truly unavoidable. You just have to endure it... Learning how to handle this stress will make you more resilient in the long run."

❹ Put Your Plan Into Action

Now that you've identified, analyzed and solved your stress, it's time to put your plan into action. Let's say you have *identified* that your long commute to work is driving you crazy. You've also analyzed it and right now you know it's unavoidable, frequent and severe.

You went through the 'solve it' step and you've come up with numerous possible solutions: you could request flex hours, move closer to work, move in the opposite direction of traffic, listen to a recorded book in the car, take public transportation, find a job closer to home, or work from home on certain days.

Now it's time to choose the solution that works best for you and put your plan into action.

Sometimes one solution just jumps off the page and is easy to put into place. But other times, you have to work out a combination of things, or get buy-in from other people like your boss. Let's say you decide the best solution is to work from home. The only problem is, you know you are going to have a hard time selling this idea to your boss.

In Tim Ferriss' excellent book, *The 4-hour Work Week*, he describes a step-by-step plan for getting your boss to allow you to work from home. He recommends that you begin by asking permission to work from home for just one day. On that day, you make sure you get about twice as much done as you usually would in the office. (Given the fact that you're saving two or more hours of commuting time, it actually might be easier than you think.) You come back to work the next day with stacks of work done and you build a case for a commuter-free life, one day at a time. (See Ferriss' book for more information on this. He will really turn your notions about how to get things done efficiently upside down.)

Look at all your possible solutions and decide which one suits your situation the best. Give yourself a deadline for putting your plan in place. Don't let fear hold you back—if you do what you've always done, *you'll get what you've always gotten*. Moving in new directions and always making course corrections when necessary will keep you *balanced*—and will help you stay at the top of the graph we talked about in Chapter 5.

www.welcoa.org ★

❺ Stay With The Plan

Identifying, analyzing and solving your stress, and then creating an action plan will help ensure that you've thought carefully about what, when, how and why you need to manage stress. As a result of taking the first four steps in this problem-solving exercise, you are light years ahead of other people who never take the time to do this. Perseverance is all you need now.

But perseverance—or staying with the plan—is a different mental muscle than all the other mental muscles you've exercised so far. Like we said back in Chapter 4, tracks have to be laid down in your brain through repetition, just as you would if you were trying to create a new path through a field of tall grass. And going back to the old path, i.e., falling off the wagon, is part of the change process.

Making your action plan part of your life plan is about living it every day. Stress really is a killer and you are taking it seriously now. You've taken all the necessary steps in order to manage it, and you just have to put the pedal to the metal and actually hold it down. Don't despair if you take some wrong turns along way. Don't let a few stressed-out days leave you feeling like you can't do it.

You Can Persevere

Stress is pervasive. It sneaks up on you when you're not looking, and sometimes over the silliest things. You're never going to be able to make yourself completely immune to it, no matter how hard you try. But every time you recommit to staying with the plan, you will further engrain your desire to stand at the top of the upside down U, maintain your balance and work at your peak.

Sure, you'll occasionally slide over the edge, but now you know how to right yourself, without completely losing your balance. You're like a surfer riding a wave of energy called stress. If you fall off that board, you know how to get back on that surfboard, paddle out against the waves and ride the next wave, and do it over and over again if necessary. *That's perseverance.*

Five Steps For Stress Management

So there you have it, the five steps for solving any stressful problem: identify it, analyze it, solve it, put your plan into action, and stay with the plan.

THE FIVE STEPS TO IDENTIFYING STRESSORS

❶ Identify It.
Take the time to keep track of your stress for a couple of weeks. You'll be surprised what you find out.

❷ Analyze It.
Think about what you've found out and determine what kind of stress it is (is it avoidable or unavoidable?), how severe it is and how frequently it occurs.

❸ Solve It.
Based on the type of stress you decide it is (avoidable, unavoidable, second-hand, anticipatory or underlying) you will have different strategies for how to solve it.

❹ Put Your Plan Into Action.
Don't let fear stop you. You know how important this is, so just do it.

❺ Stay With The Plan.
Ride the wave of stress energy and if you fall off the board, just get right back on and *go with the flow.*

> "Making your action plan part of your life plan is about living it every day. Stress really is a killer and you are taking it seriously now."

CHAPTER 8

Stress: It's Definitely My Problem To Solve

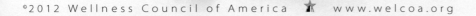

CHAPTER 8

Stress: It's Definitely My Problem To Solve

One of the first things you have to do in order to move ahead of the crowd of people who are beaten down by stress is to take ownership of your problems. Many of the stress-related problems you experience have been created by you, and therefore, can only be solved by you. This is especially true of psychological stress, which often involves faulty or overly negative thinking on your part.

Even the problems you didn't create—like getting laid-off, getting dumped by your significant other, or catching a nasty cold from a family member—are STILL YOUR PROBLEMS. When you blame other people or outside circumstances for *your* problems, you basically hand over the keys for solving that problem to somebody else.

Taking responsibility for solving your problems doesn't mean that YOU are to blame; it simply means that no matter who is to blame, you are still the one who has to solve the problem. So if you have a difficult relationship with a boss or a spouse, you can either end that relationship (if it's bad enough), or develop coping strategies like exercising or meditating daily so the stress doesn't overwhelm you. There are lots of other coping strategies and ways of handling stress, but you actually have to sit down, take ownership of the problem *first*, and then give yourself a little transition time to move into a solution-oriented way of thinking.

Shifting Your Focus Forward

Moving into a solution-oriented way of thinking requires an important process that I call *shifting your focus forward*—from the problem to the solution. Here's how it works:

When we are first confronted with a problem, the problem is all we can see. As the result of this tendency toward tunnel vision, we become *problem-oriented*. This may be due to the element of surprise coming into play (as stress often hits us from out of the blue), and because it takes us a while to adjust to our new reality (where we suddenly feel worse off than we were just seconds before when we didn't have this problem.) So it could take a few minutes, or a few hours, or even a few days to adjust to our new reality, depending on the size of the problem. While we are in this transitional phase, we often say to ourselves: *Woe is me. I have a big problem I didn't have before.*

Maybe a tree falls on your house, maybe you find out your teenager got expelled from school, maybe you didn't get the promotion you were counting on, or maybe you find out that your car needs a new transmission. In the transition phase after we FIRST hear the bad news, we tend to focus entirely on the problem which only increases our stress: *This problem is terrible; It stinks; Why does this stuff always happen to me?*

> "Taking responsibility for solving your problems doesn't mean that YOU are to blame; it simply means that no matter who is to blame, you are still the one who has to solve the problem."

> "However long it takes, remind yourself that you are moving through a transition from no longer being problem-oriented but rather becoming solution-oriented."

Making The Switch

Another reason why it's hard to move into being solution-oriented is that when we are stressed, our problem-solving ability essentially just disappears. Under pressure, especially under the intense stress you feel when you first encounter a really big problem, your 'emotional' brain (the lower part of the brain called the limbic system) takes over your 'thinking' brain (the upper cerebral cortex), and it becomes difficult to think clearly. Dan Goleman, author of the book, *Emotional Intelligence*, calls this an *'emotional highjack.'*

Imagine a moment of receiving new, disheartening information that makes you feel so angry you want to punch the wall, or yell at someone, or just scream in the stairwell. Don't expect yourself to think clearly or to do ANY form of creative problem-solving in such an agitated state. In order to move through it, you'll want to simply focus on your breathing and try to get your stress number down to a five or a four. Then you'll want to continue calming yourself down by repeating: *This is just a problem that needs to be solved.*

Depending on how good you are at calming yourself, you may need to allow a few minutes, or a few hours, or even a few days before beginning the following problem-solving exercise. However long it takes, remind yourself that you are moving through a transition from being *problem-oriented* to being *solution-oriented*. And surprisingly, this new solution orientation is sometimes all you need to make your stress number go down significantly. This happens because you will start to feel a growing sense of control over your problems.

Exercises For Becoming Solution-Oriented

Included here are five exercises you can do to help you brainstorm solutions to your stressful problems. If you're serious about managing your stress, going through these next exercises will really help.

These exercises follow the five-step program we outlined in the previous chapter and will allow you to solve many of the stressful problems you've already identified with your stress log. Write down anything that comes to mind. Silly solutions are fine because sometimes they help get your creative juices flowing and move you toward a more serious one that will actually work. Write down as many different solutions to the same problem as you can.

Throughout the process of solving the problem, quantity is almost more important than quality. The sheer number of ideas (even mediocre ones) will help spark your creativity and will help you make new connections to formulate even better solutions. It is recommended that while filling out these exercises, you sit down in a quiet room where you won't be disturbed for at least a half an hour.

SOLUTION-ORIENTED EXERCISES #1 AND #2

1 Make a list of all (or at least ten) problems you have been experiencing lately.

2 Rank the above problems from the most troublesome to the least troublesome based on frequency that the problem occurs and severity of the problem. Find the most troubling problem, put a (1) next to it and continue through your list prioritizing each problem.

(Exercises continued on next page) ▶

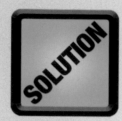
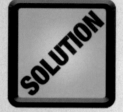
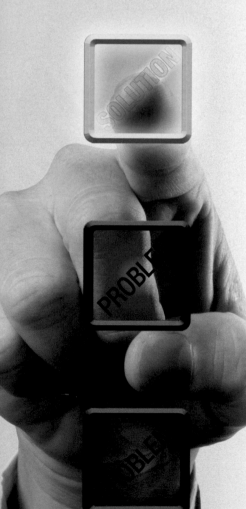

SOLUTION-ORIENTED EXERCISE #3

3 Take your top five problems. Come up with at least three possible solutions to each problem. Just keep asking yourself: *How do I solve this problem?* (Don't worry about the quality of the solutions. For now, quantity is more important than quality. If you are stumped, feel free to brainstorm with anyone you think that can offer you help.)

❶

❷

❸

❹

❺

(You may wish to allot a whole page to solving your number one problem, especially if it's a really vexing one, and devote your entire session to thinking up solutions for just this one problem. Enlist the help of a trusted non-judgmental friend, spouse, or family member if you think it will help.)

(Exercises continued on next page) ▶

SOLUTION-ORIENTED EXERCISE #4

4 Pick the problem that seems like the most pressing (or the one that you've come up with the most solutions for) and put a plan in place for dealing with it. If the solution is going to be carried out over time, put a schedule in place, too.

In order to solve this problem I need additional resources. List them here:

In order to solve this problem I am going to need help from:

I will put my plan into place by:

This problem will no longer be an issue by:

If I encounter difficulties with this problem in the future, I can always (ask for help from):

(Exercises continued on next page) ▶

SOLUTION-ORIENTED EXERCISE #5

5 Carefully define how a successful outcome of this problem would look to you. Some stressful problems will go away without a fight, but others will recur. You'll have to come up with a definition of success that allows for the occasional recurrence, but *perhaps without bothering you quite so much*. Spend some time thinking about the next few questions. They are important ones that will help guide you to the finish line.

I will consider my problem to be over when:

_____
_____
_____
_____
_____
_____
_____
_____

I know that behavioral change can involve occasional setbacks. If a setback occurs I will:

_____
_____
_____
_____
_____
_____
_____
_____

I also know that some problems (like what other people do or say) I can't control and thus may recur. I'll consider this recurrence to be OK when I can control my reaction in the following way:

_____
_____
_____
_____
_____
_____
_____

Let It Be

Sometimes you simply need to STOP thinking about your problem in order to solve it.

This approach works best with problems that come up at the end of day (and can be left until the next morning to resolve.) When this occurs at work, don't bring the problem home with you. Relax when you get home, enjoy your evening and focus on getting a good night's sleep. While you are sleeping, your brain consolidates all the input and information from the previous day and often times, when you wake up in the morning, a solution will appear that you hadn't thought of before.

You will always do better at problem-solving when you've gotten some distance from your problems and they are not staring you right in the face. If you are a morning person, try doing your problem-solving work in the morning when you're fresh and haven't been dealing with problems all day. If you're a night person, tackle this problem-solving work after you've exercised or done some other activity that takes you away from the problem and helps clear your mind.

Here's one last quote from Dr. Orman, who inspired this problem-solving approach to managing stress:

> "Everybody in life has problems, and that's what we really mean when we say we have stress. Some people, however, know how to deal with their problems better than others, **and those are the people who don't show up in my office for help with stress**."
>
> —Mort Orman, MD

CHAPTER 9

What's My Motivation?

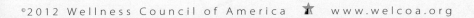

CHAPTER 9

What's
My Motivation?

Actors are famous for asking movie directors: "What's my motivation?" When it comes to wondering "what is my motivation for lowering stress?" the answers are numerous. There are so many health benefits to managing stress you'd get bored reading them all. But, the highlights include reductions in occurrences or severity of the common cold, depression, anxiety, muscle tension, chronic pain, road rage, anger, insomnia, skin rashes, digestive tract disorders, diabetes and hypertension.

Is that enough motivation?

Here's more. Take away smoking and poor diet, and stress is considered by many experts to be one of the top lifestyle risk factors for heart disease (the biggest killer by far in the US today.) And, in over 30% of cases, do you know what the FIRST sign of heart disease is?

Sudden cardiac death.

So, if stress is a risk factor in your case, you might not get ANY warning before you find out that your level of stress was TOO HIGH. Now that you know this, you probably don't want to wait to start managing your stress until it's too late. Still, we are all creatures of habit and some habits (particularly bad ones) are notoriously hard to break. Let's just accept that as a given.

If lowering your stress for a long-term health benefit isn't motivating enough, (and by the way, *for most people it isn't*), how about lowering your stress for an *immediate* benefit that you can appreciate within days? Does that sound more inspiring?

> "Take away smoking and poor diet, and stress is considered by many experts to be one of the top lifestyle risk factors for heart disease (the biggest killer by far in the US today.)"

"Your body is a storehouse for stress, which is why you go around at a much higher stress level most of the time…"

Your Total Nervous System Makeover

We've already seen what it feels like (in Chapter 1) to self-regulate your nervous system. That's an immediate benefit. And that's just a minor short-term benefit of lowering our stress levels. Now let's consider what it might be like to do a TOTAL NERVOUS SYSTEM MAKEOVER. Remember the stress scale in Chapter 1? Would a bigger investment of your time be worth it if you could wake up feeling like a 1 or 2 on the 0-10 stress number scale almost EVERY SINGLE DAY?

Your body is a storehouse for stress, which is why you go around at a much higher stress level (probably somewhere in the range of 3-5) most of the time—because you never take the time to release any steam, unwind or self-regulate your nervous system.

The Danger Of Holding It In

Let me tell you a quick story to illustrate what I mean. When I first decided to take up exercise on a 5-day a week basis, I started attending a spinning class at my local Y. (In spinning class you sit on a stationary bike and an instructor helps motivate you and your classmates to ride harder and faster.) On one particular Saturday morning, I arrived late, and the spinning instructor asked me to leave, explaining that I had not adequately warmed up.

I resisted leaving, but she was firm. It was a small insult, but I remember feeling embarrassed and angry by getting kicked out of the class in front of everyone else.

I went upstairs to another part of the facility where I could work out on an elliptical trainer. It should have been no big deal and, as you will soon see, I would have been much better off if I had immediately let my anger go. But for some reason, I didn't.

As I exercised upstairs, I remembered that the instructor would often come up after class and exercise herself. So, I decided that I was going to "give her a piece of my mind" when she arrived.

I stood hunched over my elliptical training machine, somehow holding in a lot of anger, as I worked out while waiting for her to appear. When she finally arrived, I'd been stooped over that exercise device, with my shoulders clenched, for a full 45 minutes.

She saw me, came over and apologetically explained that, for liability reasons, she had to exclude me from the class. Given the angry look on my face, I'm surprised she was willing to speak to me at all. And it was a logical, perfectly reasonable explanation for why she had to do what she did.

But the damage to my body had already been done. I had spent almost an hour on that elliptical machine feeling angry and tense. As it turned out, I'd stored enough stress in my body to last me a full month. The next day, my shoulder muscles started to spasm and this pain in my back lasted about four weeks. It took a lot of massage, numerous yoga classes, a chiropractic visit and stretching out on a foam roller to erase all the stress I stored in my muscles on that day—in less than ONE hour.

You are storing stress in this way too. Every traffic jam, every deadline, every hour you spend hunched over your computer or a steering wheel feeling frustrated, you are storing stress in your body. Without a method for releasing it, you'll start confusing a stress level of 3 *as relaxed*, and a stress level of 5 *as normal*. And that's when—if things really get stressful—you'll be more likely to escalate your internal stress levels to a 6, 7 or 8, where you may start to experience anxiety attacks and possibly even panic attacks.

Recalibrate: Get Stress Out Of Your System

So, what's your motivation for doing the exercise, stretching and meditation techniques described in this book? YOU WON'T BE STORING STRESS IN YOUR BODY. You'll be releasing it. Every day—after your stress workout—you'll recalibrate your nervous system to a 2 or a 1 or maybe even—the holy grail of stress management—zero!

Now here's my promise. Play along with me on this for at least two weeks, preferably four. I KNOW THAT'S A LONG TIME.

Let me ask you this seemingly non-related question: Have you ever had a day where, for whatever reason, you skipped brushing your teeth in the morning? How did that feel?

Not good, right? Do you need any motivation to brush your teeth? No, of course not. Avoiding that unpleasant feeling or taste in your mouth is motivation enough.

Let me tell you something amazing, but absolutely true: Now that I exercise four to five times a week, I feel so much better THAT I WILL NEVER GO BACK TO NOT EXERCISING—and I promise you'll experience a similar change. Just like you would if you skipped brushing your teeth, I get a similarly unpleasant feeling in my whole body when I skip my daily work out. (And when I miss two days in a row, I get so cranky I can't stand myself.) Talk to ANYONE who works out on a regular basis and they will all tell you the same thing— you begin to miss that easy, care-free feeling so much when you DON'T do it, that working out at least three times a week eventually REQUIRES NO WILLPOWER AT ALL!

So, your motivation here is NOT that you're going to live longer (which you probably will, by at least four years), but the REAL reason you are going to humor me and workout regularly for a couple of weeks is that you are going to feel better NOW.

In the next chapter, you'll see what you can do to release stress; to burn off steam; to get yourself to a lower stress number. To get to the other side of a good habit, you simply need to make these activities part of your daily routine—it's no different than brushing your teeth or taking a shower.

Remember one more thing, if you're an office worker, you'll spend up to 60,000 hours of your adult life sitting in a chair. Don't you owe it to yourself to spend one hour a day trying to undo all the damage your sedentary lifestyle unleashes on a body that craves physical movement, stretching and STRAIN? ⏱

"Every day—after your stress workout—you'll recalibrate your nervous system to a 2 or a 1 or maybe even—the holy grail of stress management—zero!"

CHAPTER 10

Making Stress Management Part Of Your Daily Routine

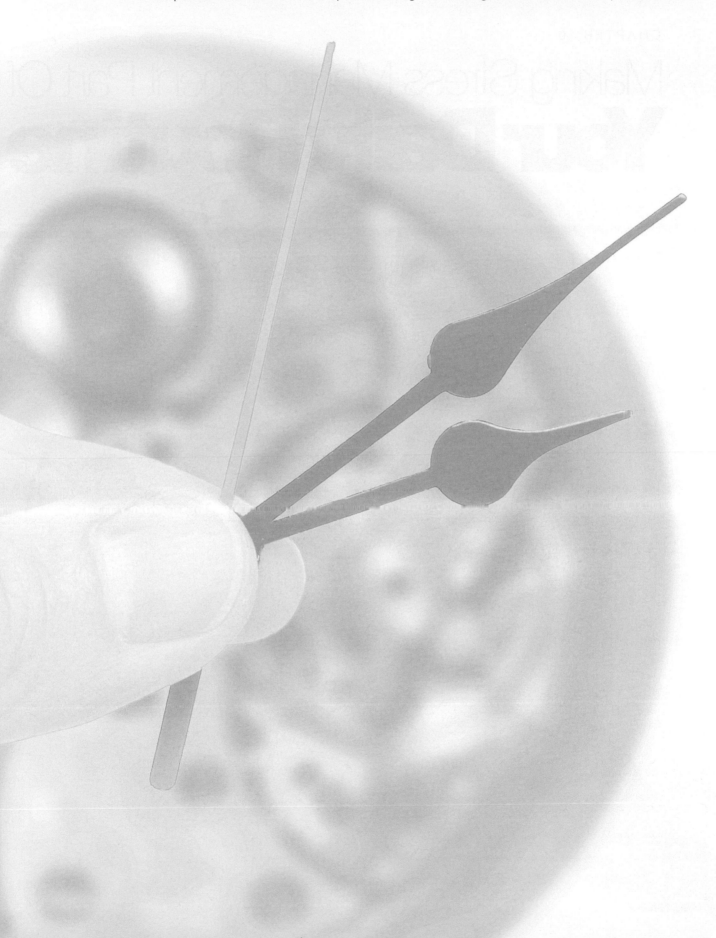

CHAPTER 10

Making Stress Management Part Of
Your Daily Routine

 www.welcoa.org ★ ©2012 Wellness Council of America

Most experts agree that time pressure is a major source of stress. That's why learning time management should be an important way to manage stress, right?

Not always. (That's the third stress management myth.)

Stephen R. Covey, author of the book, *The Seven Habits of Highly Effective People,* identified a significant flaw in the way most people manage their time. It starts with list making. If you are organized enough to actually make a list, you check things off, but somehow you never get to some of the things on your to-do list. Even on those days when you do get to most of it, you sometimes feel cheated because you'd never think of adding an hour of exercise, meditation or relaxation to this list.

In order to include a *stress management* aspect, your list should help you prioritize your tasks into those that matter most and those that matter least. In other words, you'll not only need to know what to do, but you'll also need to know *what not* to do.

Urgent, Or Important?

Covey says the problem with traditional time management all boils down to one word: URGENCY. *We get hypnotized by it.* We spend our days taking care of the *urgent (and mostly stressful)* things like putting out fires, handling interruptions, attending meetings, and answering the phone—all the while, we're *fulfilling other people's goals and dreams and not our own.* We barely EVER set aside time to do the things that WE really want to do because these activities simply aren't *urgent.*

Therefore, we often get good at doing *what matters most to other people,* but not so good at doing *what matters most to us.* Our bodies eventually wear down because we keep ignoring our own needs, which in turn affects our focus, our energy, and our enthusiasm. Without these three pillars of strength, our productivity ultimately suffers, *no matter how good we get at doing our jobs.* In order to restore our full potential, we need to devote time to our OWN wellness and our own needs—which includes finding outlets *and the time* for managing stress.

But where do we find this time?

> "Our bodies eventually wear down because we keep ignoring our own needs, which in turn affects our focus, our energy, and our enthusiasm."

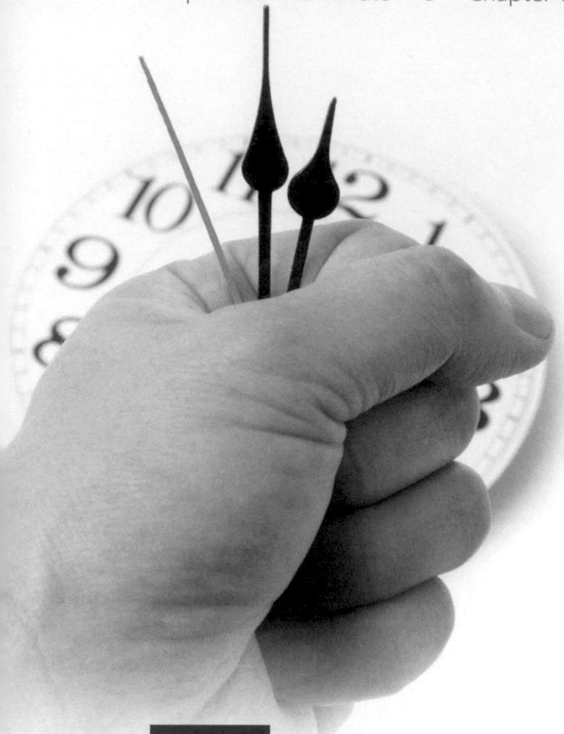

This is where Covey's Time Management Matrix can really help (see Figure 2). Using this matrix can assist you in determining what's important in your life. It's designed to help you see where you may be wasting time, or doing things that are NOT so important to YOU—or things that aren't helping you to reach your ultimate goals. Covey divides our daily tasks into four quadrants. Each quadrant is organized in terms of its urgency and importance:

Quadrant 1 tasks are *urgent* AND *important.*

Quadrant 2 tasks are *important* but NOT urgent.

Quadrant 3 tasks are *urgent* but NOT important.

Quadrant 4 tasks are *neither* urgent NOR important.

This matrix, and the simple message that it conveys, completely turned my life around over twenty years ago. But more about that after you've had a chance to study it and fully understand what it means.

FIGURE 2

Time Management Matrix

Q1: Urgent AND Important

Crises
Deadline Driven Projects
Last Minute Preparations
Medical Emergencies
Putting Out Fires

Stress

Q2: Important But NOT Urgent

Education (Reading)
Stress Management
Relationship Building
Exercise
Planning

Resilience And Personal Growth

Q3: Urgent But NOT Important

Many Interruptions
Some Phone Calls
Most Texting
Some Meetings
Watching The News

Deception

Q4: NOT Urgent And NOT Important

Surfing The Internet
Opening Junk Emails
Most TV Watching
Video Games
Computer Games

Burnout And Counter-Productive Coping

Must Do   **Should Do**   **Avoid Doing**   **Don't Do**

Quadrant 1 (Q1): *Urgent* AND *Important*:
THE QUADRANT OF STRESS

The tasks in Quadrant 1 are the ones that absolutely must get done, such as dealing with a crisis, handling medical emergencies, conducting last minute negotiations with important clients and finishing any deadline-driven project. If you spend all day in this quadrant, chances are you are going to feel stressed. If you spend *day after day* in this quadrant, chances are you are going to suffer from chronic stress and maybe even some stress-related medical conditions.

Quadrant 2 (Q2) *Important* But NOT Urgent:
THE QUADRANT OF RESILIENCE AND PERSONAL GROWTH

In this quadrant are the important tasks that we often put off because they are not urgent. Quadrant 2 activities include: exercising, taking a community college course, planning or organizing, spending quality time with loved ones and even stress management activities like meditation, yoga, or taking a relaxing, hot bath. Most people spend very little time in this quadrant because these activities aren't urgent. The less time you spend in this quadrant, the more stress you are going to experience. The main reason for this is that most of the things you do in this quadrant—from planning to organizing, exercising to meditation, or connecting with old friends to learning something new—all contribute to reducing your levels of stress.

Quadrant 3 (Q3) *Urgent* But NOT Important:
THE QUADRANT OF DECEPTION

These are the tasks that are urgent, but not necessarily important. When your cell phone rings or a text comes in, you feel obliged to answer it right away, even if you're in the middle of a lunch date with a good friend or an important client. These calls and texts are often NOT that important, but they ARE urgent.

The same is true when someone stops by your desk or work station to ask you a question, or to chat for a few minutes. It may be important to them, but it's often NOT that important to you. Never-the-less, urgency fools you into dedicating more time to these interruptions than they are probably worth. Even certain meetings that don't apply to you fall into this quadrant. Activities in this quadrant trick you into thinking you're busy and being productive when you actually aren't—and this deception ultimately leads to more stress because you're busy doing things that don't contribute to your ultimate goals in life.

Quadrant 4 (Q4) *Neither* Urgent NOR Important:
THE QUADRANT OF BURNOUT AND COUNTER-PRODUCTIVE COPING

These are the tasks that are neither urgent nor important. This is usually the stuff we do at the end of the day (or sometimes in the middle of the day if we are really burned out) that are often a complete waste of time. These activities include surfing the internet, opening junk mail, reading every email, making personal calls at work, watching TV, or playing computer and video games when you get home. Often times we spend precious minutes or even hours in this quadrant trying to recover from all the time we've spent in Quadrant 1!

> "Covey's Time Management Matrix divides our daily tasks into four quadrants. Each quadrant is organized in terms of its urgency and importance."

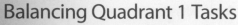

Balancing Quadrant 1 Tasks

When you analyze this quadrant it's easy to see that these are the tasks that just have to get done. The urgency associated with completing Quadrant 1 tasks may make you feel stressed, but it will give you a heightened sense of pride and accomplishment when you are able to meet these stressful challenges head-on. And, as we said earlier, what helps you manage these stressful challenges is the planning, exercise, yoga and meditation you do in Quadrant 2. Just remember, you don't want to spend all your time in Quadrant 1 because eventually that will lead to burnout.

Making Time For Quadrant 2 Tasks

Quadrant 2 activities get put off because they are not urgent. Daily planning, for example, is rarely urgent. You can always skip it if you don't have time. But when you do skip it, you're likely to spend even more time in Quadrant 1 cleaning up the messes that were created by your LACK of planning. Sometimes referred to as "the tyranny of the urgent," Quadrant 1 activities always SEEM more important than Quadrant 2, and thus, inevitably succeed at getting our attention first. But, if we spend all our days doing nothing but urgent things we will never develop and grow as human beings. We will never reach our full potential. We'll never become what Covey calls a *highly effective human being*.

So how do we find time to dedicate to these *important* Quadrant 2 activities?

Simple. We steal time from Quadrant 4 and dedicate it to Quadrant 2. This is how I completely turned my life around over twenty years ago.

Making The Switch

I wanted more time to exercise and manage my stress—and to learn about stress management and ultimately write about it. But where was I supposed to find this time? I had a full time job and a family to support. It took many months of nearly falling asleep while reading bedtime stories to my young children (between 8:00 and 9:00 PM) before it dawned on me: *why don't I just go to bed around the same time as my kids?* Then I could wake up earlier and put the time to good use in the morning. At first the idea of forgoing all my favorite late night TV shows really seemed like a major sacrifice: *what about Monday Night Football? What about the 11 o'clock news? What about Jay Leno?* Despite my reservations, I decided to give it a try. After all, those TV shows were all Quadrant 4 activities.

It took me a few days to adjust to the new schedule, but soon I was waking up around 4:00 or 5:00 AM feeling fully rested and ready to start my day. Now I had 2-3 hours of completely uninterrupted time to write, exercise, read and/or do yoga. I had stolen 2-3 hours from my Quadrant 4 activities and successfully converted them into Quadrant 2 activities, which up until that moment, I never had the time to do before. Everything that I've managed to create today—including my business, my lifestyle, the roof over my head and THIS VERY BOOK that you are holding in YOUR hands— was conceived and grown out of this ONE SIMPLE STRATEGY.

Target Your Time-Wasters

Look at your life, and ask yourself where are you spending time (the currency of your life) that you could redirect elsewhere?

TV is an easy target. Americans watch on average five to six hours of TV a DAY! But even if you're not a big TV-watcher, there are other time-wasters you can target, too. I used to think that reading the newspaper every morning was a high-priority task. And for a while, I was a news-junkie—reading two newspapers, listening to news radio in the car and watching CNN on TV—thinking, *oh no, I couldn't possibly give up the news. How am I supposed to keep up with world events?* Now, I set limits. I read a news magazine once a week and check out certain major breaking stories on the internet, but I stay on top of things just about as well as I did before.

Ever played solitaire on your computer? I used to do the timed-version where you get bonus points for playing quickly. I was completely hooked on it and would play for at least an hour EVERY DAY. It was my escape (a mild form of counter-productive coping.) But, one day I just stopped because, in addition to being a TOTAL waste of time, it was not relaxing at all. It was raising my adrenaline levels instead of lowering them. (And why not use that time to do something REALLY relaxing?)

I noticed the same thing was true about watching football and baseball games. It wasn't relaxing. I could feel my adrenaline levels rise as the game got more exciting. If my team won, there was great rejoicing. But if my team lost, or something else disturbed me while I was watching it (like my kids knocking over the popcorn bowl), I was much more likely to snap at them or be crabby, or just be frustrated by the whole experience. As the result of this observation, I still watch sports, but not nearly as much as I used to. I find it quite satisfying now to turn a game on more towards the end and just watch the last hour or so.

> "Another key teaching point of The Time Management Matrix is that URGENCY often fools us into NOT doing the things that are really important in life."

Stress Management 101: Repurposing Your Time

Look for easy targets—the tasks or activities where you are clearly spending a lot of time in Quadrant 4—and repurpose this time for something more productive such as reading or learning something new, or spending time with your family, or even doing something really relaxing like taking a hot bath or engaging in your favorite hobby. Whatever it is you do—try to make it something truly rejuvenating. Another key teaching point of the Time Management Matrix is that URGENCY often fools us into NOT doing the things that are really important in life. We always think the urgent things are more important than the non-urgent things. You might be the next Hemingway or Steinbeck who's about to write the Great American Novel, BUT when your mobile phone rings, you answer it right away because it's urgent and therefore seems more important.

Don't let this happen to you. As Covey recommends, try setting aside 60 to 90-minute blocks of time in your schedule every day, where you know you won't be interrupted. Whether it's first thing in the morning like I did, or some other time of day that works better for you, here's the most important thing:

> *Whatever time you have set aside for doing your important tasks—like exercising, meditating, doing yoga, or reading something educational or inspirational—don't let any seemingly urgent task (especially those deceptive ones from Quadrant 3) knock you off of your regular schedule.*

(That's why first thing in the morning worked so well for me, because almost no one is going to interrupt you at 4:00 AM. *Even small children sleep later than that.*)

Scheduling Quadrant 2 Activities

Now let's talk about when you are going to *schedule* your Quadrant 2 activities.

(For a sample list and calendar you can use, please see Figure 3.) Remember, taking the time to actually write these activities into the schedule on the following page increases your commitment to them, and increases the likelihood that you will actually do them and make them apart of your daily routine.

Use the sample list of activities and calendar in Figure 3 to make up your own time-management plan for moving Quadrant 2 activities into your daily routine. Your list should include the important tasks and stress management activities that you want to spend more time doing. You can select from this list, or create your own list.

Deep Breathing (2 min.)	Listening To Music (10 min.)
Progressive Muscle Relaxation (5 min.)	Reading (30 min.)
Yoga Stretches (10 min.)	Massage (30 min.)
Yoga Class (60 min.)	Nap (20 min.)
Meditation (20 min.)	Walk (10-30 min.)
Exercise (20 min.)	Planning Your Day (15 min.)
Hot Bath (20 min.)	Organizing Your Workspace (30 min.)

FIGURE 3

Quadrant 2 Activities

	SUN	MON	TUE	WED	THU	FRI	SAT
5–6 AM							
6–7							
7–8							
8–9							
9–10							
10–11							
11–12							
12–1 PM							
1–2							
2–3							
3–4							
4–5							
5–6							
6–7							
7–8							
8–9							
9–10							
10–11							
11–12							

If you work a normal daytime shift, the gray areas in the sample calendar represent times that might be available for doing your Quadrant 2 activities. You should decide how you want to fill in these shaded time slots. Do you want to rearrange your whole day, like I did, by going to bed earlier and getting up earlier (*When you won't be interrupted?*) Or, would you rather choose certain time slots that were formerly taken up by Quadrant 4 activities and reschedule your new Quadrant 2 activities in there?

It's fine to start small. Just 15 minutes a day of exercising or meditation is a great place to start. That way you can establish a habit and build on it.

By looking at the list of Quadrant 2 activities, notice how in little more than a half an hour, you could squeeze in five minutes of progressive muscle relaxation, two minutes of deep breathing, 10 minutes of yoga stretches and 20 minutes of exercise. You would undoubtedly be a completely different person if you dedicated JUST this amount of time to your health and well-being every day. Think about the benefits of starting your day with this modest regimen—you'd lower your stress number and would be more likely to maintain a lower average number throughout the day, (since as we've learned, our stress hormone levels tend to build from whatever baseline we establish at the beginning of the day.)

Sticktoitiveness

Remember that doing your Quadrant 2 activities will require some willpower and resolve. Because studies show that willpower tends to wane as the day progresses, here again, it might be better for you to do these activities in the morning, if you can. (But there's no reason why you can't do them later in the day, just as long as you don't let any Quadrant 1 or Quadrant 4 activities steal this time away from you.)

The Take-Away

There's an old saying that we mentioned in Chapter 4 : "first you make your habits and then your habits make you." This inspiring bit of wisdom may be the very thing that nudges you over the threshold and causes you to schedule your very first activity that's wholly devoted to managing your stress. Think very carefully about the schedule that YOU are going to create, look at the Quadrant 4 activities you can eliminate and commit yourself to this new schedule for at least a couple of weeks.

Here's the take-away from this chapter: You don't have to ADD stress management activities to your already over-burdened schedule: You literally have to TAKE AWAY something first. Then you will be replacing an activity that's not so vital to your health and well-being with something that is— even though it might not be urgent. Eventually, if you make the time to include any combination of these stress management activities as part of your day, *they will become habits*—no different than brushing your teeth or taking a shower.

We have now shattered three myths about stress management. Can you remember the third one? If so, write it down.

....

....

....

....

....

Hint: Time management always helps you manage stress. True or false??

"You don't have to ADD stress management activities to your already over-burdened schedule: You literally have to TAKE AWAY something first."

EPILOGUE

Stop Stress This Minute
In Summary

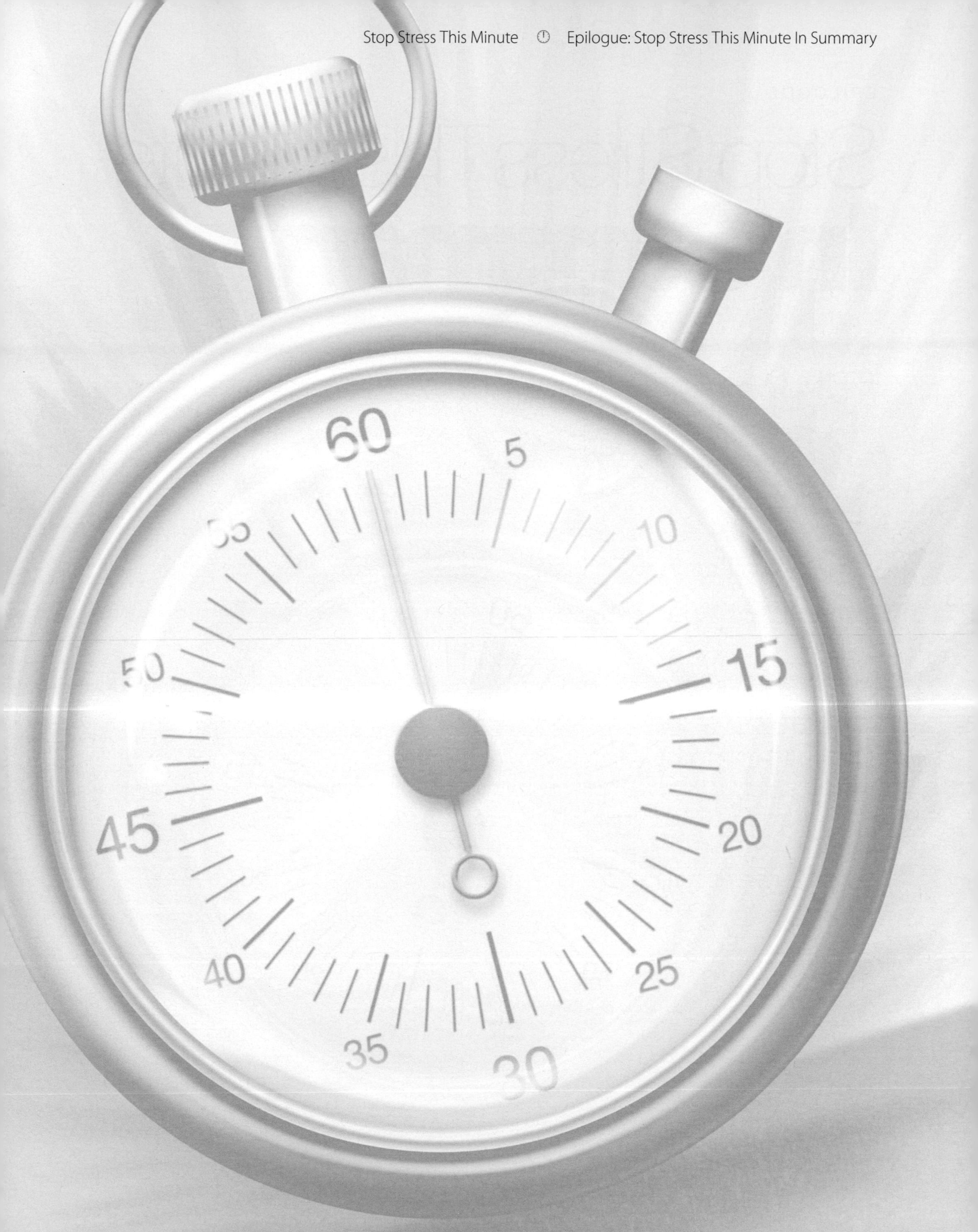
60
5
10
15
20
25
30
35
40
45
50

EPILOGUE

Stop Stress This Minute
In Summary

S cientific research confirms that having stress outlets and a sense of control are critical when it comes to managing stress. This research, conducted on rats, showed that when a rat feels more in control of its stress or has an outlet for managing that stress, it will fare much better than a rat that doesn't. As long as this rat has a lever it can press to control the stress, or outlets for releasing the stress like a running wheel to jump on or a piece of wood to gnaw on—it is much less likely to develop ulcers and other stress-related complications than the rat that doesn't have those things.

Your Controls And Outlets

In this book, we've tried to give you numerous options for controlling your stress and/or finding outlets for managing it. In the first two chapters, we gave you ten ways to stop your stress in just minutes. These quick and easy methods include deep breathing, progressive muscle relaxation, meditation, jumping rope or climbing stairs, and/or stretching.

In chapters three and four, we talked about how your thinking can be a major source of stress. We gave you five ways to change it, including: 1) learning to dispute your overly negative thoughts; 2) becoming aware of how judgments cause YOU stress; 3) limiting your worry to times when you can actually DO something about it; 4) learning to accept what is and can't be changed; and 5) keeping your stress in perspective.

In chapters five and six, we narrowed in on the addictive behaviors you have to change—the classic counter-productive coping trap of overeating, overspending and drinking   in order to manage your stress. We showed you how to change such addictive behaviors by moving through what psychologist James Prochaska calls the stages of change—knowing exactly *what* you want to change, and outlining *why* you want to change and *how* to go about changing—before you even BEGIN to think about actually *making* a change.

In chapters seven and eight, we pointed out that problem-*solving* is one of the best forms of stress management. Instead of seeing our lives as filled with stress—which might seem unsolvable—it would be better off if we could break our stress down into specific problems, most of which, on an individual basis, can be solved quite readily. We showed you a simple five-step method for solving stressful problems, which included analyzing and breaking down your stress into different types such as avoidable and unavoidable stress.

In chapter nine, we looked at motivation. Just improving your health as it turns out, for most people, isn't motivation enough to help them make permanent lifestyle changes. In order to effect lifestyle change, you need to make stress management a part of your daily routine, much like brushing your teeth or taking a shower. When you think about how you feel when you DON'T brush your teeth or take a shower, you realize that these activities *require no motivation at all*—and a similar thing happens when you exercise and manage stress on a daily basis.

And finally in chapter ten, we showed you how to use Stephen Covey's Time Management Matrix to carve out the time you need to do important stress management activities such as exercise, yoga and meditation on a daily basis, while understanding how *urgent* tasks can fool you into skipping these *life-affirming* activities.

So, Stop Stress—Right This Minute

Please, don't use lack of time as an excuse for not managing your stress and consequently NOT realizing your full potential as a human being. The Covey matrix is designed to help you find the time, but even if it doesn't, there are so many things that we have shown you that can help you manage stress in little or no time at all:

1. Deep breathing takes less than a minute and will significantly lower your stress.

2. Changing your thinking requires no time at all and faulty thinking may be the biggest source of stress of all.

3. Counter-productive coping always costs you time in the long run. Deciding to change your addictive and counter-productive behaviors requires plenty of willpower, but it takes no time—*it only saves time.*

4. When you start looking at stress as simply a problem that needs to be solved, the job of managing your stress becomes so much clearer and so *doable.* This approach requires about an hour a week where you sit down and do some plain, old-fashioned problem-solving.

5. You can easily trade an hour of TV-watching each day for an hour of exercise, meditation, or yoga (or any combination thereof.) Once you make these IMPORTANT Quadrant 2 activities a part of your daily routine, that hour will be the most important hour of your day.

When you say, *I don't have enough time to manage my stress,* what you really may be saying is *I don't want to manage my stress.* Or *I'm not worthy.* Or *my health is NOT that important to me.* Or *it interferes with what I perceive to be more important goals.* Or *I don't value my peace of mind.* Please don't kid yourself. It's not about the time. It's about you and what you TRULY value in life. Your health is important—and there's no more important goal than feeling good inside because it affects EVERYTHING and EVERYONE with whom you come in contact.

Your happiness *and productivity* depend on this internal source of good feeling. It's way more important than anything you might accomplish by spending an extra stressed-out hour at work. The hour you devote to working out or managing stress RECHARGES your batteries, while the extra hour you spend at work simply drains them.

Start now. You just have to set aside the time every day and commit to the program for long enough (we're talking about a couple of months) to get to this magical point where your efforts require virtually no motivation at all. Where the desire to do these things springs from the way you feel inside.

Feel Well And Be Well—Every Day

I want you to wake up feeling well and be well every day: *this is your birthright*. To see a child skipping across a parking lot and know in your heart that you feel like skipping too—to live lightly on the earth, to be happy to be alive, to live with optimism instead of pessimism and to be grateful instead of ungrateful.

Keep in mind, the goal here is not a stress-free life. The goal instead, is to provide you with outlets and solutions for *managing* your stress so that you can maintain your equilibrium despite whatever stress may come your way. Make no mistake about it: *I still get stressed out by life circumstances both big and small.* And truth be told, on most days I wake up feeling just a little bit anxious.

Why?

There are two reasons: 1) Cortisol levels (a stress hormone) are naturally at their highest in the morning. I can clearly feel this when I first awaken; and 2) Anxiety runs in my family and I've been a bit anxious my whole life.

That's why I NEED this stuff. That's why I take it so seriously. And that's why on most days, the first thing I do is a half hour of *vigorous aerobic exercise*. I usually follow that with at least 20 minutes of yoga, which I conclude with a meditative rest period of about 10 minutes. What you do may be completely different from what I do, but with those three practices under my belt, I can easily reset my nervous system to a 1 or 2 on most days. (On some days, I can even get down to zero.) And that peaceful beginning usually stays with me for the whole day.

I can't live without that hour of stress management on most mornings. And I can almost guarantee that once you incorporate this stress management hour into your daily schedule, you won't be able to live without it either.

Please set aside time to manage your stress. As you nurture and grow that peaceful place inside you, you will have the great pleasure of passing this peace of mind forward from person to person to person. Share a smile with everyone you meet and provide a listening ear and a reassuring word to the people you interact with and *you will feel more at ease and more at peace*.

By lowering *your* stress, you can lower *other people's* stress too. And by lowering other people's stress it lowers your stress, yet again. It's a remarkable, but very real neurological phenomenon—*and this phenomenon makes stress management not just a gift that you give to yourself, but one that you share with the whole world.* ☺

MY TOP 5 METHODS FOR REDUCING STRESS

Your top five may be completely different from mine, but here's what works for me and why:

1. **Vigorous Exercise.** I personally work out almost every day. Exercise is such a reliable way to manage my stress that I always recommend it to other people. (Talk to your doctor before starting ANY exercise program.)

2. **Yoga.** Think of the word flexible—that's how you want to feel both mentally and physically.

3. **Meditate.** This is a hard one for a lot of people, including me. My mind often goes a mile a minute when I meditate—but over time I've found it helps me feel more decisive, less fearful and more patient.

4. **Talk therapy.** Talking to a friend or a therapist is a delightfully easy way to reduce stress. Look for a non-judgmental friend you trust who you can talk to on a regular basis. I am fortunate to have a friend like this and we talk for about an hour each week.

5. **Organize and plan.** When my life gets disorganized, I get stressed. It's as simple as that. 15 minutes a day of planning and one day a month of organizing really makes a noticeable difference for me.

In total, I devote close to an hour a day to managing my stress. But remember, if you're just starting out, start small. 15 minutes a day doing any of the techniques in this book is a great place to begin.

Resources And References

Chapter 1

Doctor visits for stress-related conditions: Rosch, Paul, MD, "America's #1 Health Problem,"(see: www.stress.org)

Stress-related diseases: Rosch, Paul, MD, "Effects of Stress," (see: www.stress.org)

Side effects: "Study Links Smoking Drug to Cardiac Problems," New York Times, July 5, 2011.

Masking symptoms of stress: "Are Acid Reflux Drugs Overused?" (see: WebMD.com)

0-10 Stress measurement is commonly used to measure pain: "Pain Education Video Appears Effective in Whiplash Treatment," Journal of the American Psychological Association, February 2007, Vol. 38 No. 2.

Meditators at Harvard: Benson, Herbert, MD, "The Relaxation Response: How to Counteract the Harmful Effects of Stress," Lecture at Wesleyan University, May 25, 2007, (see: www.Wesleyan.edu/alumni/weseminars)

Fight or flight: Benson, Herbert, MD, "The Relaxation Response," p. 54-56.

Interview with Dr. Martin Samuels: Ballantyne, Coco, "Can a Person Be Scared to Death?" (see: www.ScientificAmerican.com)

Voodoo death: Rosch, Paul, MD, "Sudden Death and Heart Attacks." American Institute of Stress Newsletter, August 2006.

Stress recovery time: Goleman, Daniel, PhD, "Social Intelligence," p. 232.

Stress is cumulative: Goleman, Daniel, PhD, "Emotional Intelligence," p. 61.

Chapter 2

The effects of meditation: Benson, Herbert, MD, "The Relaxation Response," p. 110-118.

Breathing frequency: Fried, Robert, PhD, "Breathe Well, Be Well," p. 29.

Measuring breath: Joan Borysenko, PhD, "Minding the Body, Mending the Mind," p. 64.

Progressive muscle relaxation: Gessel, Arnold H., MD, "Edmund Jacobson, MD, PhD: The Founder of Scientific Relaxation," International Journal Of Psychosomatics, Vol. 36(1-4), 1989.

Benefits of yoga: Benson, Herbert, MD, and Eileen Stuart, R.N., "The Wellness Book," p. 79.

Lower blood pressure by listening: Lynch, James, PhD, "Interview with James Lynch;" University of Minnesota Website (see: http://takingcharge.csh.umn.edu)

Attunement: Goleman, Daniel, PhD, "Social Intelligence," p. 25.

Attention span: on web BBC News, "Turning Into Digital Goldfish," February 2002, (see: http://news.bbc.co.uk)

Benefits of meditation: Ornish, Dean, MD, "The Spectrum," pp. 122-123.

Brain research: Sapolsky, Robert, PhD, "Stress and Your Body," pp. 314-315.

How to meditate: Benson, Herbert, MD, "The Relaxation Response," pp. 170-173.

Guided imagery: Naparstek, Belleruth, "What is Guided Imagery?" and "Three Principles of Guided Imagery," (see: www.healthjourneys.com)

Altered states: Benson, Herbert, MD, "The Relaxation Response," pp. 125-126.

Effects of deep relaxation: Benson, Herbert, MD, "The Relaxation Response," pp. 110-118.

Effects of exercise on stress: Ratey, John, MD, "Spark," pp. 57-84.

Chapter 3

Ranking stress: American Psychological Association: "APA Survey Finds Rising Stress Takes a Toll," 2007, (see: www.apapracticecentral.org/update/2007/10-25/stress-survey)

Origins of cognitive psychology: Abrams, Mike, PhD, "A Brief Biography of Albert Ellis," (see: www.rebt.ws/albertellisbiography.html)

Ellis vs. Beck: Ellis, Albert, PhD, "All Out," p. 456.

Awfulizing, etc.: Ellis, Albert, PhD, "How to Keep People From Pushing Your Buttons," pp. 29-31.

Effectiveness of cognitive therapy vs. medications: "Cognitive Therapy vs. Medications for Depression: Treatment Outcomes and Neural Mechanisms," (see: http://www.ncbi.nlm.nih.gov)

ABCs: Ellis, Albert, PhD, "How to Keep People From Pushing Your Buttons," pp. 7-20.

Space between stimulus and response: Covey, Stephen, PhD, "The 8th Habit," p. 42.

Chapter 4

On cognitive restructuring: Carey, Benedict, "Working Long Hours? Take a Massage Break, Courtesy of Your Boss," The New York Times, September 7, 2004.

Henry Ford quote: (see: www.goodreads.com)

Neuroplasticity: Siegel, Daniel, MD, "Mindsight," pp. 5, 42.

Thinking about thinking: Ellis, Albert, PhD, "How to Stubbornly Refuse to Make Yourself Miserable about Anything, Yes, Anything," p. 14.

I can't stand it: Ellis, Albert, PhD, "How to Stubbornly Refuse to Make Yourself Miserable about Anything, Yes, Anything," p. 147-149.

Unwritten rules: Beck, Aaron, MD, "Love is Never Enough."

Rhinehold Neibhur: Goldstien, Laurie, "Serenity Prayer Skeptic Now Credits Neibhur," The New York Times, November 28, 2009.

Neurons in the gut: Siegel, Daniel, MD, "Mindsight," pp. 5, 43.

Stress is funny: LaRoche, Loretta, "The Joy of Stress," Video, WGBH Educational Foundation.

Misery index: Jasheway, Leigh Anne, "Don't Get Mad, Get Funny!" pp. 47-50.

Chapter 5

Stress and optimal performance graph: Goleman, Daniel, PhD, "Social Intelligence," pp. 270-271.

Hans Selye: Orman, Mort, MD, "The 14-Day Stress Cure," p. 2.

N.I.C.E. stress: Eliot, Robert, MD, "From Stress to Strength," p. 45.

Counter-productive coping: Snow, David, PhD, "Coping with Work and Family Stress," Handout 1.4.

Addiction: Greene, Bob, "Don't Sleep with Your Cell-phone Nearby," November 1, 2011, (see: CNN.com)

Behavioral addictions: Frances, Allen, MD, "DSM5 Suggests Opening the Door to Behavioral Addictions," March 24, 2010, (see: www.psychologytoday.com)

TV-addiction: "Television and Health" (see: www.csun.edu, The Sourcebook For Teaching Science)

Effects of stress: Sapolsky, Robert, PhD, "Why Zebras Don't Get Ulcers," pp. 13-14.

Chapter 6

Stages of change: Hartney, Elizabeth, "The Stages of Change Model in Addiction Treatment," (see: www.About.com Guide) Updated July 13, 2011.

Relapse and stress: Prochaska, James, PhD, "Helping Populations Progress Through the Stages of Change," (webcast, see: www.bu.edu)

Modeling bad behavior: "Use of Cigarettes by Preschoolers While Role-Playing as Adults," (see: http://hoodcenter.dartmouth.edu)

Not ready for action: Prochaska, James, PhD, "The Trans-Theoretical Model," (see: http://www.prochange.com/ttm)

Abstinence violation effect: Siegel, Ronald, PsyD, "The Mindfulness Solution," p. 262.

Chapter 7

Stress as problem-solving: Orman, Mort, MD, "The Secrets Of Dealing With Stress: A Live Radio Interview With Dr. Mort Orman, MD," (see: www.stresscure.com)

Underlying causes of stress: Orman, Mort, MD, "The 14 Day Stress Cure," pp. 17-24.

Anticipatory stress: Saplosky, Robert, PhD, "Why Zebras Don't Get Ulcers," pp. 6-7.

Working from home: Ferriss, Tim, "The 4-Hour Work Week." pp. 210-225.

Chapter 8

Emotional hijack: Goleman, Daniel, PhD, "Emotional Intelligence," pp. 13-14.

Unconscious mind consolidates memories while we sleep: "Sleep, Learning and Memory," (see: http://healthysleep.med.harvard.edu)

Stress as problem-solving: Orman, Mort, MD, "The Secrets Of Dealing With Stress: A Live Radio Interview With Dr. Mort Orman, MD," (see: www.stresscure.com)

Chapter 9

Risk Factors for heart disease: "Heart Disease: Risk Factors," (see: www.Mayoclinic.com)

Living longer with exercise: "How Can Exercise and Diet Make You Live Longer?," June 14, 2010, (see: www.Livestrong.com)

60,000 hours of sitting: "Sedentary Adults," (see: beactive.com.au)

Chapter 10

To-do lists: Covey, Stephen, PhD, "The 7 Habits of Highly Effective People," pp. 149-151.

Time management matrix: Covey, Stephen, PhD "The 7 Habits of Highly Effective People" p. 151.

Tyranny of the urgent: Covey, Stephen, PhD "The 7 Habits of Highly Effective People" p. 146.

TV time: "Television Statistics," (see: www.csun.edu)

Setting aside time for Quadrant 2 activities: Covey, Stephen, PhD "The 7 Habits of Highly Effective People," pp. 333-340.

Willpower: Tice, Dianne, "How Can We Get Willpower Back Once it Has Been Depleted?," (see: www.science andreligiontoday.com)

Epilogue

Research on rats: Sapolsky, Robert, PhD, "Why Zebras Don't Get Ulcers," pp. 255-256.

Cortisol levels spike in the morning: Naiman, Rubin, PhD, "Healing Night," p. 121.

Emotions are contagious: Goleman, Daniel, Ph.D., "Social Intelligence," pp. 108-109.

Stop Stress This Minute: Stress Journal

DATE/TIME	INCIDENT	DESCRIPTION

Stop Stress This Minute: Stress Journal

DATE/TIME	INCIDENT	DESCRIPTION

Stop Stress This Minute: Stress Journal

DATE/TIME	INCIDENT	DESCRIPTION

Stop Stress This Minute: Stress Journal

DATE/TIME	INCIDENT	DESCRIPTION

Stop Stress This Minute: Stress Journal

DATE/TIME	INCIDENT	DESCRIPTION

Stop Stress This Minute: Stress Journal

DATE/TIME	INCIDENT	DESCRIPTION

Stop Stress This Minute: Stress Journal

DATE/TIME	INCIDENT	DESCRIPTION